YOGA FOR LIFE

HOW TO STAY STRONG, FLEXIBLE & BALANCED OVER 40

JOSEPHINE FAIRLEY

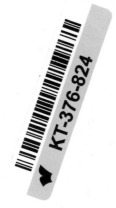

PHOTOGRAPHY BY CLAIRE RICHARDSON

KYLE BOOKS

DEDICATION

To all the wonderful yoga teachers who have helped me on my journey: Simon Low, Godfrey Devereux, Liz Lark, Hilary Totah, Romana Balle, Chris Elam, Lisa Powell, Stephanie Shanti, Hayley North and Fiona Livingstone. Om shanti.

613.7046

First published in Great Britain in 2012 by
Kyle Books
an imprint of Kyle Cathie Limited
23, Howland Street
London W1T 4AY
general.enquiries@kylebooks.com
www.kylebooks.com

ISBN: 978 0 85783 043 2

A CIP catalogue record for this title is available from the British Library

Josephine Fairley is hereby identified as the author of this work in accordance with Section 77 of the Copyright, Designs and Patents Act 1988

Text © Josephine Fairley 2012
Photography © Claire Richardson 2012 except pages 8–9, 22–3, 215 © Corbis; pages 21, 145, 198–9, 206–7, 213, 217 © Getty Images; pages 203 and 209 © istock and pages 210–11 © Lotus Journeys
Design © Kyle Books 2012

Editor: Vicky Orchard
Design: Debi Angel
Photography: Claire Richardson
Copy editor: Susannah Marriott
Production: Gemma John and Nic Jones

Colour reproduction by Scanhouse in Malaysia
Printed and bound by Toppan Leefung Printing Ltd in China

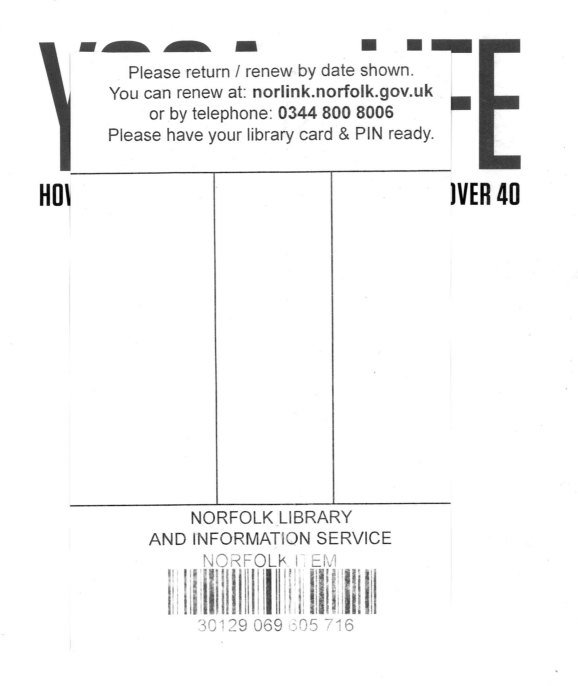

HOW VER 40

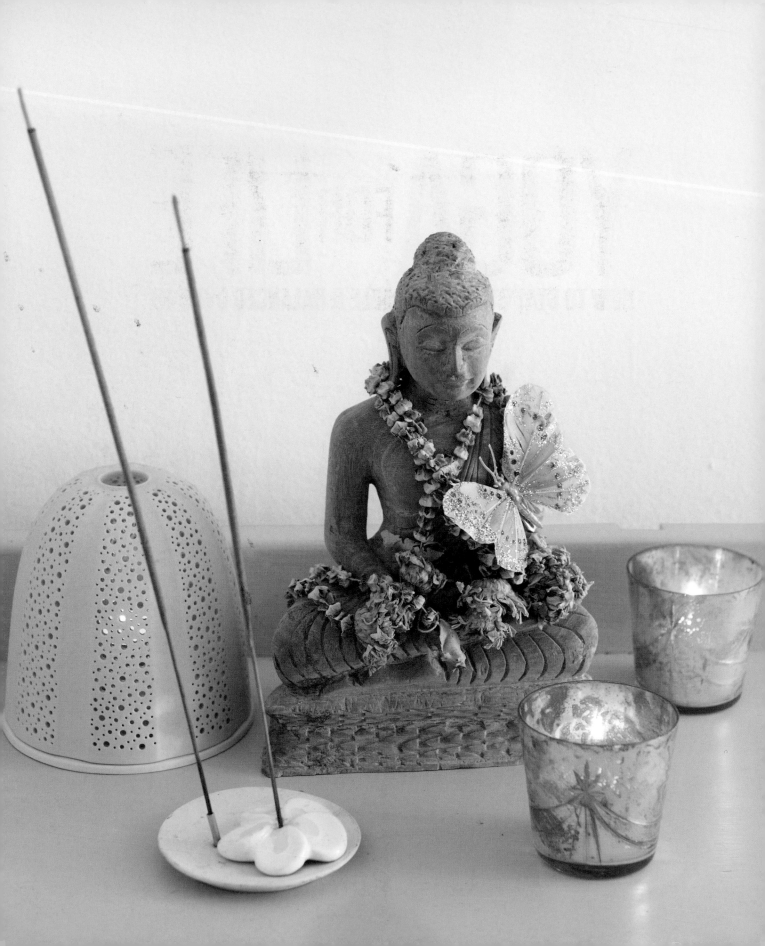

CONTENTS

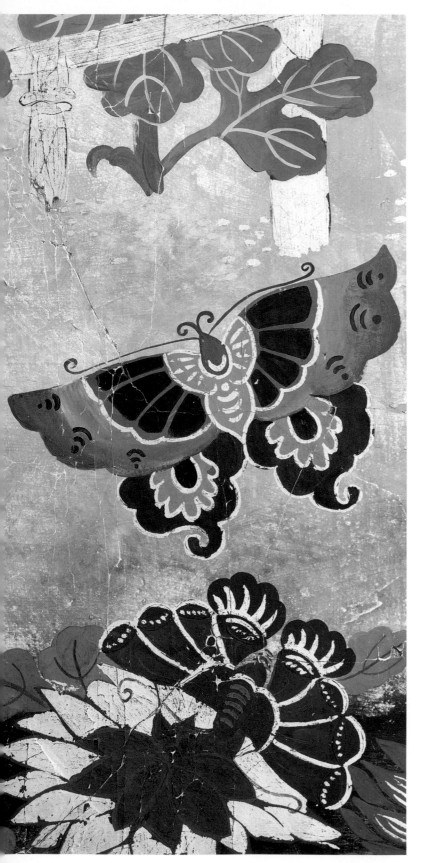

It was in Los Angeles that I first met Jo Fairley, over 25 years ago – in a Hollywood rock club on Sunset Boulevard, watching the rhythm and blues artist Robert Cray. She shared my love of music, chocolate, and later, quite clearly, yoga. By the time we met again Jo had opened a wellness centre in Hastings, on the south coast of England. Yoga is an offering central to her establishment's wellness programme: it is a practice at the very heart of wellness.

After a colourful, stressful and successful life of hard work and hard play in the music industry in London and New York, I discovered yoga in my early 30s. I never remember having stretched before, let alone taken a conscious breath. I was a perfect candidate for yoga, and the yoga I was offered was perfectly pitched. It gave me the inner strength and awareness to take responsibility for my health and healing, and is now the source of my healthier life and livelihood. Yoga not only gave me much improved posture and mobility, it taught me methods for self-healing after years of debilitating lower-back pain, poor digestion and breathing, (I suffered from asthma as a child), while also giving me a broader perspective on life and its potential. Now as a full-time yoga teacher, a large number of my students in all of the many countries I visit to teach are over 40, and many are still practising yoga regularly and enjoying a healthy active life in their 80s and 90s. It is never too late, or too early to start yoga. Equally, it is never too late to enjoy its numerous and well-documented benefits.

As an anchor for the mind during the skillful and focused exploration of the many shapes and sequences of contemporary yoga, the physical

FOREWORD
by Simon Low

practices and positions (asanas) have been well documented to provide improved flexibility and strength, stamina, proprioception and circulation, conscious breathing, healthy and mobile joints, and enhanced concentration and awareness. My anatomy and physiology studies, alongside my own yoga experience, suggest that not a single cell is left untouched by the influence and energy of yoga, and not an area of our lives is left unaffected.

Yoga is a tool for life. A fuller, finer, fitter life. It stimulates the very essence of life, the animating energy of prana, yoga's term for 'life force', most easily accessed through *pranayama*, the conscious breathing practices that support and surround all of our physical postures, whether flowing or still, active or passive, strong or soft.

The classroom can indeed frequently become a physically challenging environment for the yoga body – especially that with a few more laps under its belt. In more recent years, the perception fostered by the celebrity-obsessed media is that yoga is for the young, athletic and body beautiful. The most common comment I hear when I ask people if they are interested in trying yoga is that they are not flexible enough, or cannot do yoga because they could not possibly manage to get into *padmasana*, the lotus pose, (an advanced sitting position with a leg configuration that only a small percentage of yoga practitioners should ever even attempt until many years of careful practice toward the required hip flexibility is achieved). Another common reason people do not take up yoga is a fear that their injuries or ailments would be worsened.

My first teacher, Larry Payne, to whom I will forever be grateful for so graciously sharing yoga's ancient wisdom and healing potential – would always remind those fortunate students who attended his classes in west Los Angeles that yoga should be accessible and appropriate to the individual, and encouraged personal responsibility toward the safe and effective practice of postures to honour our unique bodies. It was this emphasis on the individual's needs, balanced with the appropriate application of effort and ongoing commitment, that was to shape my life and eventually my teaching.

Needless to say, skillful anatomically aware teaching is an essential prerequisite for safe teaching, and those who have chosen to try yoga, and take the time to find the right teacher, and the approach that resonates with them are most often rewarded with a life-long friend in yoga, and soon realise that with a good teacher and the appropriate class level or style, they can not only 'do yoga' but enjoy and benefit from its gifts regardless of age, condition or experience. Yoga is for everyone, everywhere. If you can breathe you can practise yoga.

In my classroom a teenage newcomer 'mats up' next to a senior student, whether senior in age or experience. Yoga does not discriminate. Yoga is for life, and for living, and offers a happier and healthier life for students of any age, physical condition, culture or creed. This book is a welcome addition to the yoga bookshelf as it opens its pages to embrace all those who wish to learn yoga from the beginning, with gentleness, care and simplicity, without dumbing down, over-simplifying or underestimating yoga's practice, progress or potential.

www.simonlow.com
www.theyogaacademy.org

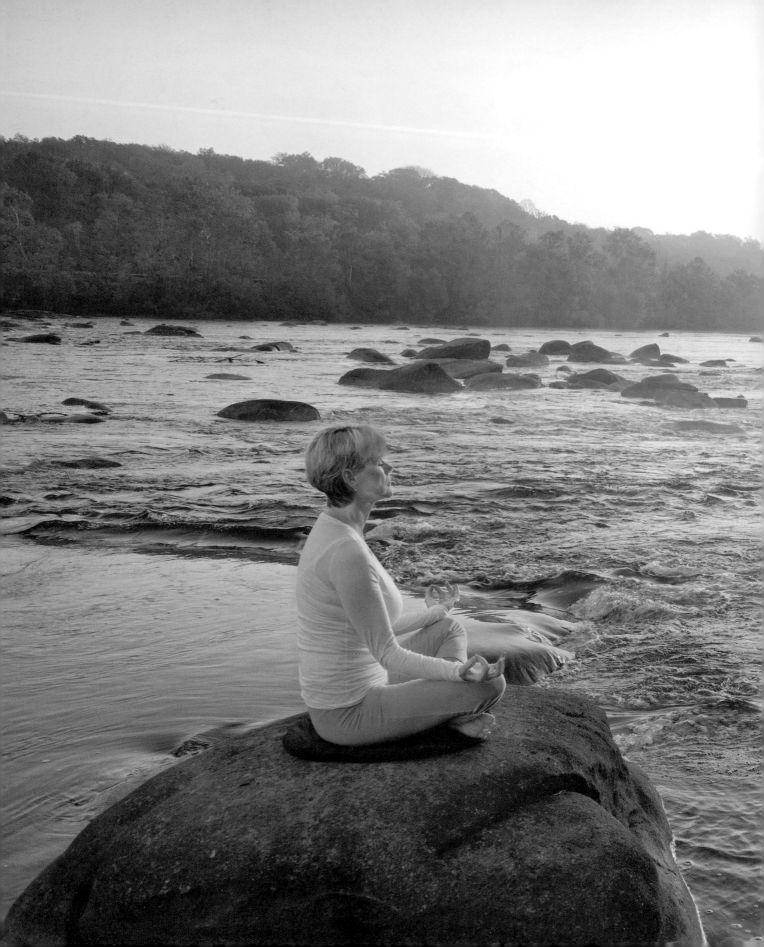

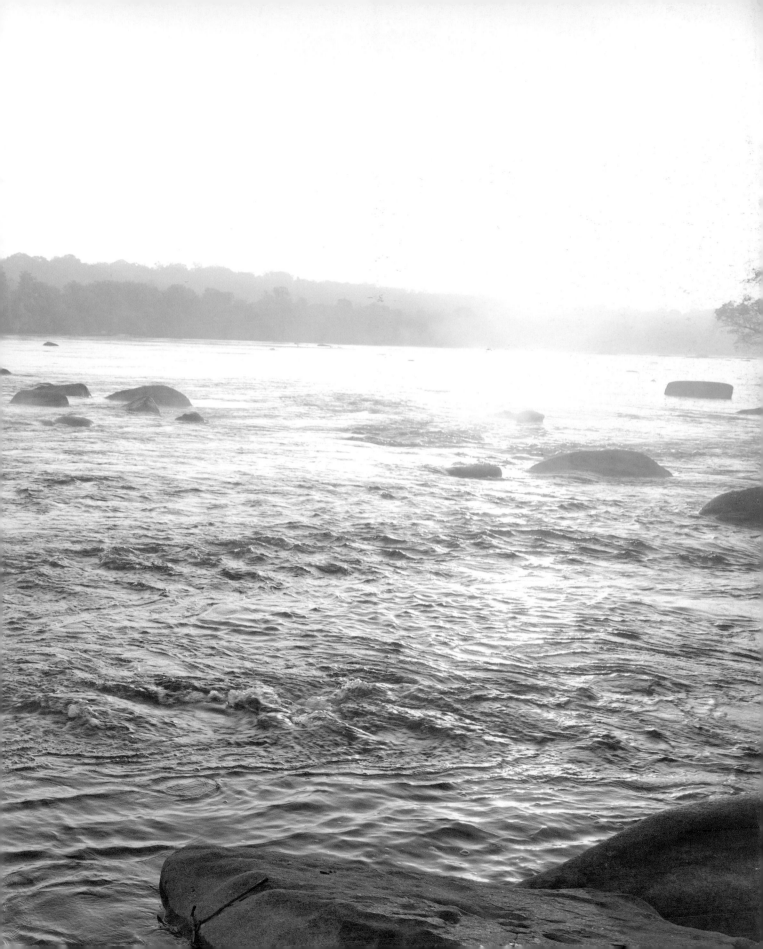

INTRODUCTION

As the author of several books on how to keep ageing at bay, I tend to give one simple, nugget-sized piece of advice to the countless people who ask me every year for my 'ultimate anti-ageing secret'. It is, quite simply, 'Take up yoga.'

As far as I am concerned, yoga is literally the fountain of youth. I have seen fabulous, flexible seventy-somethings practising yoga: sharp of jaw, super-flexible, admirably strong. I contrast them to the 'little old ladies' – of a similar age, if not younger – who can be seen tottering precariously down the streets. I've seen fabulous older men, too, standing upright, shoulders back, able to touch, well, if not their toes, then at least their insteps.

I am just one of millions of individuals outside India – where yoga was born – to understand that in my busy and stressful Western life, many aspects of yoga help me to cope with everything life throws at me. And it can do that for you, too. Countless studies are emerging which show that yoga is good for everything from balancing hormones to improving flexibility (so that if you do fall over later in life, at least the landing is softer).

I've dipped in and out of yoga all my life, but it wasn't till I was in my 40s that I started really to understand what it does for me – and to make sure that I wove it into the fabric of my days. I've introduced more friends than I can count to yoga, too – and each of them, at some point, has told me how it's changed their life, too. How they wish they'd known about it earlier, they say, now they are so much less stressed, more energetic and able to roll with life's punches.

Yoga has been an amazingly supportive friend to me over the years. It's something I have turned to when I've felt unable to cope, and it's helped me to re-ground myself and get my life back in balance. Twice, it's saved me from falling apart when I was faced with enormous challenges – one a bad road accident, another a true-life tragedy. Instead of wailing or screaming or panicking, I stood tall, did some yoga breathing and centred myself. I was able to think crystal-clearly and to cope.

Five years ago, after selling my interest in Green & Black's – the chocolate company I started with my husband, Craig Sams – I had the chance to invest in something else I really believed in, again in partnership with my husband. There were two ventures to fill in the missing pieces of our local 'healthy-living jigsaw'. The first was a one-stop organic and local bakery-cum-foodstore almost on our doorstep. The second venture – and this is where yoga comes in – was a well-being centre with a beautiful, L-shaped room. Walking into the near-derelict ex-council building, it was the possibility of a yoga studio that gave me goosebumps. I could see the potential, and somehow, I knew that room was going to become an important part of my life.

I road-tested yoga teachers, adding to the roll call of dozens of others I've tried over the years (and I've 'kissed a few frogs' en route to my perfect yoga teachers). I went to workshops, to glean insight into how other people had set

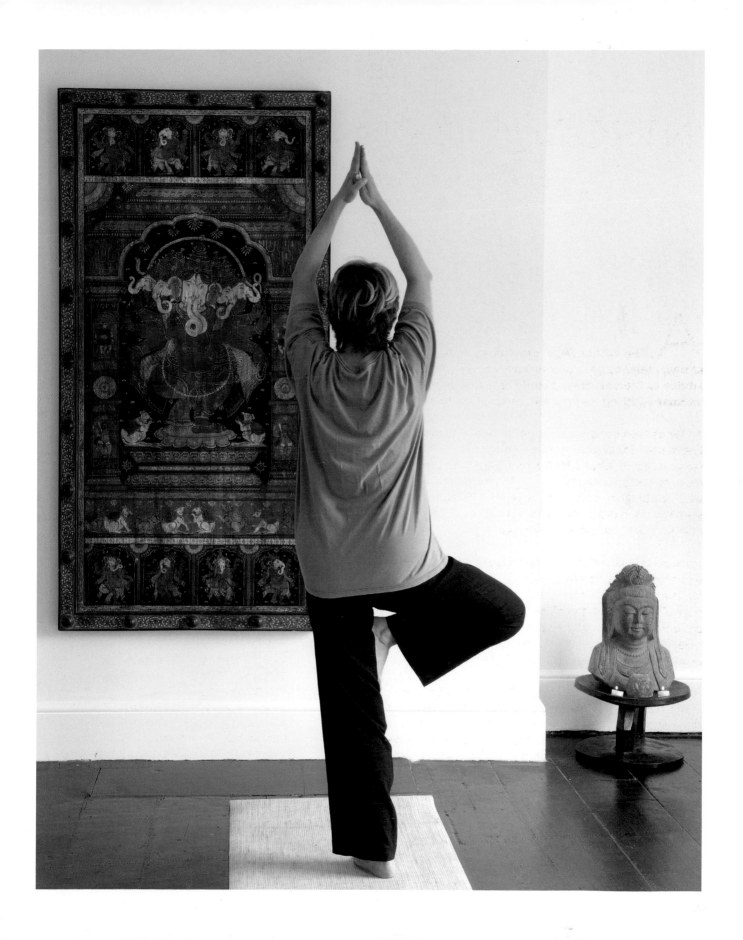

about creating the perfect space in which to practise yoga. I started to go on 'yoga vacations' (or at least to places where yoga was an activity option), which deepened my knowledge and ironed out a few mental kinks along the way. And finally, I got the hang of how to integrate yoga into my daily life at home, so that now each morning I start the day not only with a cup of English Breakfast, but also a few hip rolls and some Downward Dogs, at the very least. And my day is all the better for it. In fact, the days when I don't do at least some yoga seem to unravel pretty fast.

At 'my' studio – at The Wellington Centre in Hastings, East Sussex – I've now watched, over the past five years, many other people's lives being transformed by regular yoga. It's a fact that the studio tends to attract many slightly more mature students – at least in the classes I pitch up for regularly. Among the regulars is the woman whose hip pain has completely disappeared following a couple of years of yoga (she'd been on painkillers up to that point). There's the early-morning-yoga friend whose crippling migraines are history, which she also puts down to yoga. I've also seen several women with 'body issues' – generally, shyness about carrying too much weight – who've felt stronger and more positive about themselves after starting yoga, and have escaped the spiral of 'comfort eating'. So while the weight hasn't fallen off the way it would with a crash diet, because they're thinking 'mindfully' – including eating mindfully - they've almost effortlessly shed a few pounds and transformed their relationship with their bodies and with food.

Over the years, I've built up a pretty comprehensive bookshelf of yoga books. All of them are written by yoga teachers. So as a yoga 'consumer', they didn't always tell me what I needed to know: how to find the perfect teacher, buy the right kit and get back on the mat when I've lost my yoga mojo.

Whatever I've done – whether it's starting a chocolate company, writing a beauty book, opening a bakery or creating a wellness centre – I have put myself in my customer's shoes first and foremost. And that's where I'm standing right now (if you can be barefoot on a yoga mat *and* wearing a customer's shoes…). So while this book lays out the yoga postures – asanas – that are most helpful from mid-life onwards, leading you through them individually (and as sequences), it also has all the stuff I think that people want to know about yoga for mid-life and beyond (with expert input from yoga teachers I know and respect).

Of course you can read this book if you're 20-something and new to yoga. But really, it is for anyone who's 40-plus, and who may be fresh to yoga or wants a yoga practice that's right for this stage in life. It's for individuals who go to classes and studios, and for those who prefer an at-home yoga practice. It's also for those of us who like a spiritual dimension to their yoga, but prefer to avoid some of the 'mumbo-jumbo' that often attaches itself to this ancient practice.

But whoever you are, and at whatever stage of life you happen upon this book, my intention is for it to help you make yoga part of your life. For a lifetime.

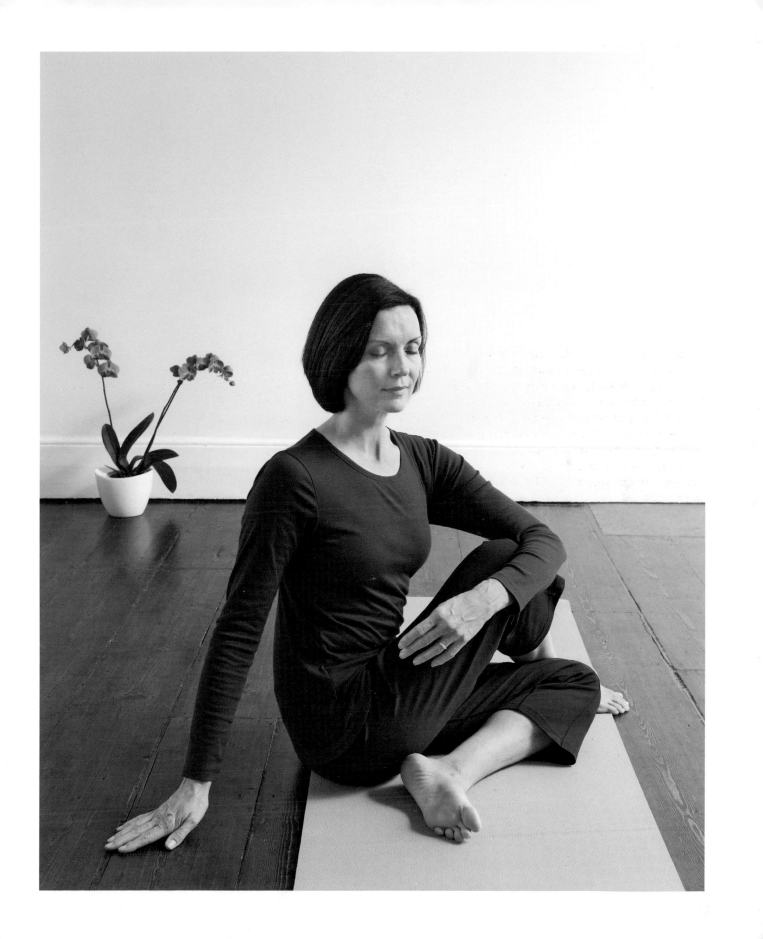

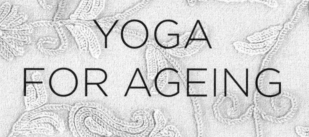

CHAPTER ONE

YOGA
FOR AGEING

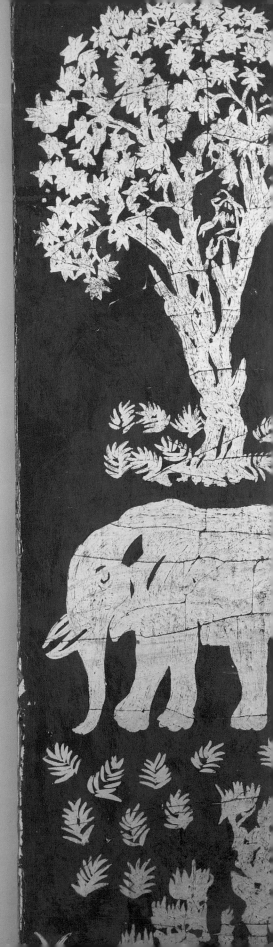

Don't know about you, but I have absolutely zero desire to become one of those little old ladies leaning on a walking stick. Z-e-r-o. Let alone a Zimmer frame. Even when I'm 103.

And as far as I am concerned, one of the key ways to prevent a frail body is, quite simply, regular yoga. So it is rather gratifying that studies around the world are, increasingly, confirming that yoga can help fight all manner of challenges that face our ageing bodies (not to mention minds): loss of bone density, stiffness (of the brain, too), hardening of the arteries, hormonal fluctuations, mild depression....

The list is pretty endless, but here are some of the key reasons why yoga is so darned fah-bu-lous for older bodies. Sure, it's great when you're 20 and want a flat, show-offable stomach, but multiply 20 by two or three or more, and the benefits are exponentially greater. As Dr. Friedrich Staebler, a doctor/acupuncturist/herbalist, has observed, 'People understand their cars better than their bodies. If we get a new car, we assume it will work without trouble for a while, then things will begin to wear and need attention. It is the same with the body. If we give it the right attention when needed, rather than ignoring it and hoping it will go away, our body need not be a source of pain and discomfort.'

It is, frankly, never too late to take up yoga. (Although never too early, either.) In one study, for the University of California, Los Angeles (UCLA) School of Medicine, 21 people who were aged 60 or over started to take a yoga class twice a week. They all had rounded backs – that dreaded 'dowager's hump' – which can interfere with normal movement. And the measured benefits were really impressive. The curvatures themselves were reduced by 6 per cent, walking speeds were upped by 8 per cent, and the 'reaches' of the volunteers in the study improved by 18 per cent. What's more, many of the volunteers reported that their balance had improved, as a side-benefit.

The study, published in the *American Journal of Public Health* (AJPH), suggested that the yoga produced an increase in overall strength and flexibility. (Though frankly, anyone who's done yoga even for a little while could have told them that...). Added the researchers, 'The contemplative state encouraged by Yoga's mind-body approach may also lead to enhanced well-being, a benefit noted by the majority of our participants.'

'Yoga transforms a negative approach to life into a positive one.
It helps us take care of ourselves at a time of need.
Daily practice of yoga will keep old age at bay'

BKS Iyengar

YOGA FOR SPECIFIC PROBLEMS

Specific sequences of yoga postures can benefit all sorts of aches, pains and stiffness, as well as problems like mild depression, which can become more common with the passing years. Later in the book, I'll list some postures that may be helpful if you have certain physical challenges, as well as 'the blues' (see pages 168–72).

Many of us who spend time at computers, for instance, have wrist problems – in some cases, leading to carpal tunnel syndrome (CTS), in which swollen tendons press on the wrist. Typically, a conventional medical approach is to immobilise the joints with splints, or even turn to surgery to reduce compression. But another positive study – published in the *Journal of the American Medical Association* (JAMA) – showed that for mild symptoms, yoga can again be incredibly effective. Researchers found that CTS sufferers who did Iyengar yoga twice a week for eight weeks experienced a four-fold improvement in grip strength and a two-fold reduction in pain, compared to their be-splinted peers. You can read more about this form of yoga – which stresses proper alignment – on page 32, though my hunch is that virtually any gentle form of yoga would have shown similar results. Yoga helps with circulation – especially in the hands and feet.

As someone who used to have freezing-cold extremities throughout the winter, I've experienced this first-hand – and, er, first-feet. Yoga boosts blood flow to cells, which function better as a result. Twisting postures, in particular, are great for 'squeezing' blood out from the internal organs, encouraging oxygenated blood to flow once you release the twist. Inverted postures are good because they encourage blood to flow from the legs and pelvis back towards the heart, where it's freshly oxygenated before being pumped out again. That's why yoga can be very beneficial if you have swollen legs or even kidney problems. It's also been found to lower 'bad' (LDL) cholesterol and raise 'good' (HDL) cholesterol,

as well as lowering blood sugar. Oh, and did I say that yoga is effective for bringing down high blood pressure? And for stress? It reduces levels of cortisol, which the adrenal glands produce when we face challenging situations.

Yoga is also great for your bones. Osteoporosis is one of the big worries as we age, with the prospect of vertebrae collapsing (leading to the aforementioned dowager's hump, not to mention terrible pain), or even bones 'snapping' to trigger a fall. And as experts learn more about yoga, we gain more evidence that yoga – and in particular, yoga plus a plant-based diet – boosts bone health. Yoga is a form of weight-bearing exercise, which is what we're told we need more of to keep our bones healthy: resisting gravity puts a mild 'stress' on the bones, which has the effect of encouraging them to lay down more growth. Jogging, walking and playing tennis are also weight-bearing exercise – but yoga doesn't wear down cartilage or stress the joints.

A small pilot study on bone loss and yoga in 2009 enrolled 18 people who had osteoporosis or osteopenia (its precursor). After a baseline bone density test at the start, seven people were assigned to the control group, and 11 learned a ten-posture yoga sequence. Poses were maintained for at least 20–30 seconds, and the whole routine took ten minutes or so. Two years later, both groups' progress was checked and further bone scans undertaken. Although almost every member of the control group either lost bone or maintained their status quo, around 85 per cent of the yoga group gained bone in the spine and the hip. The results were published in the journal *Topics in Geriatric Rehabilitation* – and blew away the doctor who carried out the study. 'I was shocked at the results,' commented Dr. Loren Fishman. 'By putting tremendous pressure on the bones without harming the joints, yoga may be the answer to osteoporosis.' Wowzer. Dr. Fishman has since written a whole book on the subject that is worth checking out: *Yoga for Osteoporosis* (see page 221).

To get a good idea of your correct alignment find a corner of a wall and line up your head and spine with the edge, with feet placed flat either side

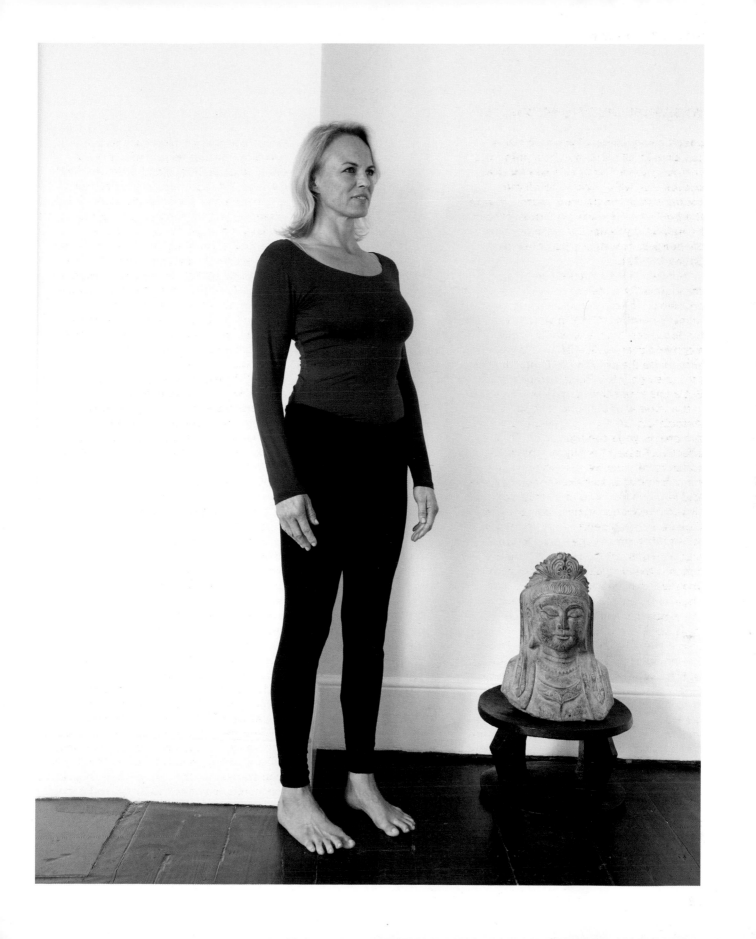

YOGA FOR A LONG LIFE

There may be yet another way that yoga is linked with longevity - and that's to do with its famous ability to strengthen our abdominal muscles. OK, at a certain age, maybe you're not going to have a pancake-flat stomach even if you do yoga several times a week. (Yoga works on the underlying abdominal muscles, making them strong and flexible, rather than delivering the 'six-pack' effect.) But think on this: as part of a very widespread Canadian Fitness Survey, 8,116 individuals were assessed. Upper body strength, grip strength and general flexibility appeared to have no effect on how long individuals lived - but those with weaker abs had a higher death rate than the rest of the group. No matter how much weight they carried around the waist.

Yoga also helps us simply to accept ourselves as we grow older, and feel better about our bodies, even when they're not perfect. As clinical psychologist and yoga practitioner Janeen Locker observes, 'Body image has to do with how you feel in your body, how you describe your body and how you think people perceive you.' What yoga does, experts believe, is help us to 'disengage' from judging our bodies, allowing us simply to experience them. And over time, that makes us feel more positive about our body image. And it is hard not to become rather pleased with your body when you find that you are able to balance almost effortlessly in Tree Pose, or open your hips wide for a forward bend, or even reach your toes for the first time! Yoga is a practice that fosters in us a more familiar, intimate relationship with our bodies by teaching us how they function. It's true: we may never have a 'perfect' physique like Christy Turlington, no matter how long we practice yoga. But (this is a slightly un-yogic thought), I'd put money on you feeling 100 per cent better about your body, whatever its shape, weight or size, after practising yoga for a while. It is simply something that happens. I have never met anyone who doesn't feel 'more comfortable in his or her skin' (as the French say), after practising yoga.

BUT IS YOGA ENOUGH?

Despite all the many benefits of yoga listed here, I'm not suggesting that yoga is the only form of exercise that anyone should do. A combination of yoga and brisk walking, to get the heart pumping and the lungs working, seems to me to be the optimum approach to healthy exercise. The American Council on Exercise (ACE) agrees: in trials they carried out, yoga (Pilates, too) fell short of the physiological markers considered necessary for a workout to be labelled an 'all-over' workout. As Dr. Gary Brickley, a senior lecturer in exercise physiology at the University of Brighton, notes, 'Basically, you need to sweat and push yourself progressively harder to improve fitness.'

There are some yoga classes that promise this – Bikram, or 'hotbox' yoga, or really dynamic forms of yoga such as Astanga. You can find more about these styles of yoga on pages 32–5. But can I just say this? If you're a beginner, or anything but the most experienced of mature yoga students, Don't Go There. The more dynamic forms are really not the place to start a yoga practice. You might think you're killing two birds with one stone, but you're quite likely to do yourself an injury trying to keep up with a fast-paced, sweaty class of much younger people. Get your cardio exercise from walking, speed-walking or swimming, but not from a punishing, power-yoga-style workout.

This book features a run-down of simple, do-able postures that you can slip into at home. But I can't recommend highly enough that you also find a class to go to. A good teacher will inspire you and help you to identify which are the best postures for you. And that hour, or hour-and-a-half, on the mat – away from distractions, the siren call of the laundry basket and the demands of friends and family – will, I promise, be an oasis in your day. Besides, you probably own a shelf full of cookbooks. But does that mean you never eat in a restaurant?

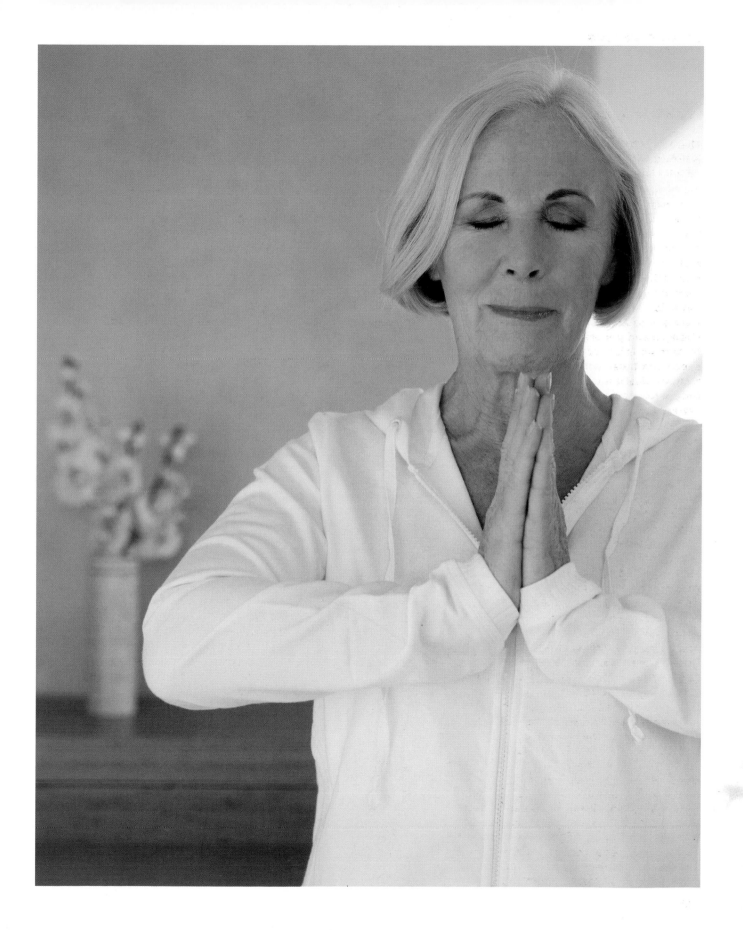

YOGA FOR LIFE'S CHANGES

Most women find themselves on a physical and emotional rollercoaster in the run-up to menopause. This time of upheaval is often marked by night sweats, weight settling around the middle, mood swings and even, sometimes, depression. Yoga can be a great support at this time as at all times of crisis or change – and so here are my top tips:

- **Breathe through it** Try 'conscious breathing' for menopausal symptoms such as hot flushes. A study published in *Menopause*, the journal of the North American Menopause Society, found that 15 minutes of simple breathing exercises (or pranayama) practised twice a day cut hot flushes by up to 44 per cent. I actually know women who've banished their menopausal symptoms entirely through regular yoga: the symptoms literally disappeared. For some breathing techniques, see Chapter 8.
- **Forget Astanga yoga, for now** Astanga (see page 32) is popular because it's fast-paced, dynamic, super-strengthening and can flatten tummies and melt away pounds. However, it builds up heat in the body and many women find that worsens hot flushes.
- **Don't even consider Bikram yoga** This much talked-about 'hotbox' method is taught in a heated room. If you're experiencing the inner inferno effect of hot flushes, my hunch is that this is probably the last place you'd want to spend time.
- **Position yourself near an open window** Whether in class or during your home practice, choose a spot near a window or door whenever possible. Some teachers prefer to keep windows shut, but if you find this physically difficult – because of hot flushes - do have a discreet word since yoga really can build body heat effectively. During the relaxation at the end of your practice it can help to shut the window, however, because the body cools down very swiftly when lying still.

Yoga can be a fantastic support during perimenopause or the change of life

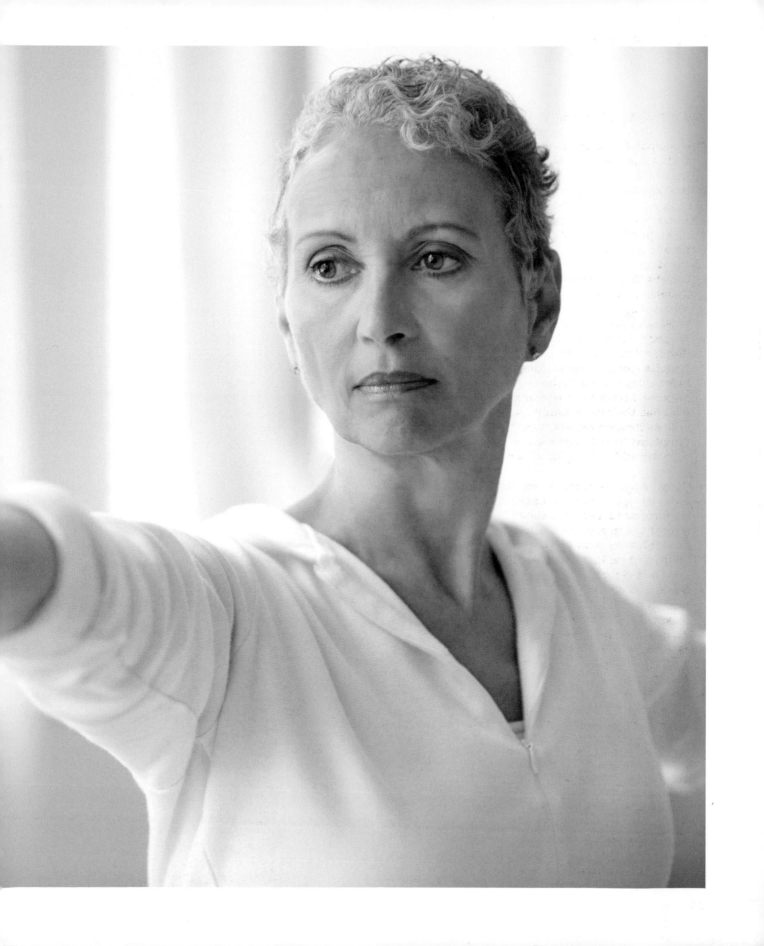

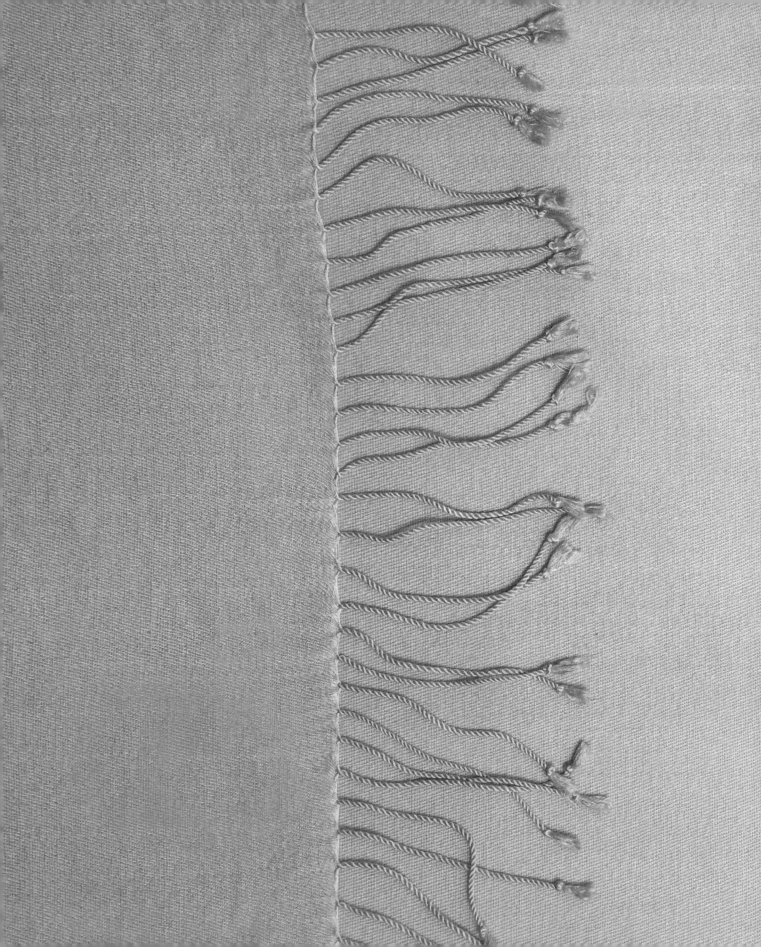

CHAPTER TWO

FINDING YOUR
PERFECT TEACHER

This book leads you gently by the hand through many different yoga poses that are useful and often highly enjoyable for women and men who are 40-plus. (And indeed, beginners of any age.) However, although it's certainly perfectly possible to explore the world of yoga with the help of a book and without ever crossing the threshold of a yoga centre or draughty village hall, there really is nothing like a class to deepen your practice.

Trust me, it's all about the teacher, and you may have to kiss a few frogs before finding your yogic prince or princess. When you do make that connection with the right person – when you just 'click' with a teacher – it can transform your experience, opening your eyes to aspects of yoga you've never thought about before. Quite possibly, it will also open your hips that bit further at the same time. I've done dozens of different classes over the years, in dozens of different locations. Some I've loved, some I've hated, but here's what I've learned:

'When the student is ready, the teacher will come'

Buddhist proverb

TALK TO THE TEACHER

Most yoga classes are advertised with the teacher's mobile number on the flyer. If you don't already know someone who goes to the class, call the teacher beforehand so that you can establish whether the poses are held for a length of time or whether you move swiftly from one to another, and whether chanting or meditation are involved. I have one friend who is almost physically allergic to the 'spiritual' side of yoga and I can feel her anger rising if she's asked to chant so much as a single 'om'. If you, too, don't give a fig for yoga's spiritual side, you may also find yourself irritated by a class that focuses on the meditative elements, rather than giving you the physical workout you're looking for. You can save yourself a lot of grief by establishing this beforehand. Although the truly 'yogic' approach would be to give everything a go, keep an open mind and see what unfolds.

Sometimes, the best class is on your doorstep In reality, few of us are going to go very far out of our way – at least, on a regular basis – to get to class, and (as with home practice) it is the regular practice of yoga that makes all the difference in the world. So, while there may be a completely brilliant teacher on the other side of town, it may work better for you to find someone closer to home or your workplace. This teacher may only be OK (not stellar), but it's often better to accept that rather than stress yourself by driving or taking public transport to a class further away, for which you may often end up being late. Yoga, as we're repeatedly told, is all about acceptance. (Though being seriously unhappy with a teacher or a setting is never acceptable.)

Ask friends for recommendations This is such an obvious point, but have you? This tip is not always foolproof, but makes a good place to start the search for your perfect yogi.

Avoid yoga at a gym If the yoga class on your doorstep is at a gym, my advice would be to think twice about making this your regular class. Many gym-based yoga teachers are former aerobics or fitness trainers who've done a yoga weekend course or module rather than in-depth training. In addition, though it's completely against the spirit of yoga, I've found gym yoga classes to be more competitive than other classes – you may feel tempted to push yourself further than is comfortable to 'keep up'. Bad idea.

Check out the teacher's qualifications It can be hard to 'unravel' a yoga teacher's credentials because there are so many different traditions, and training can vary from a weekend workshop to years of study. But no teacher should feel offended if you ask about his or her qualifications before you take a class. Unless a teacher of local classes comes personally recommended, that's the best course of action. Then you can check out online what the qualification entailed. Information

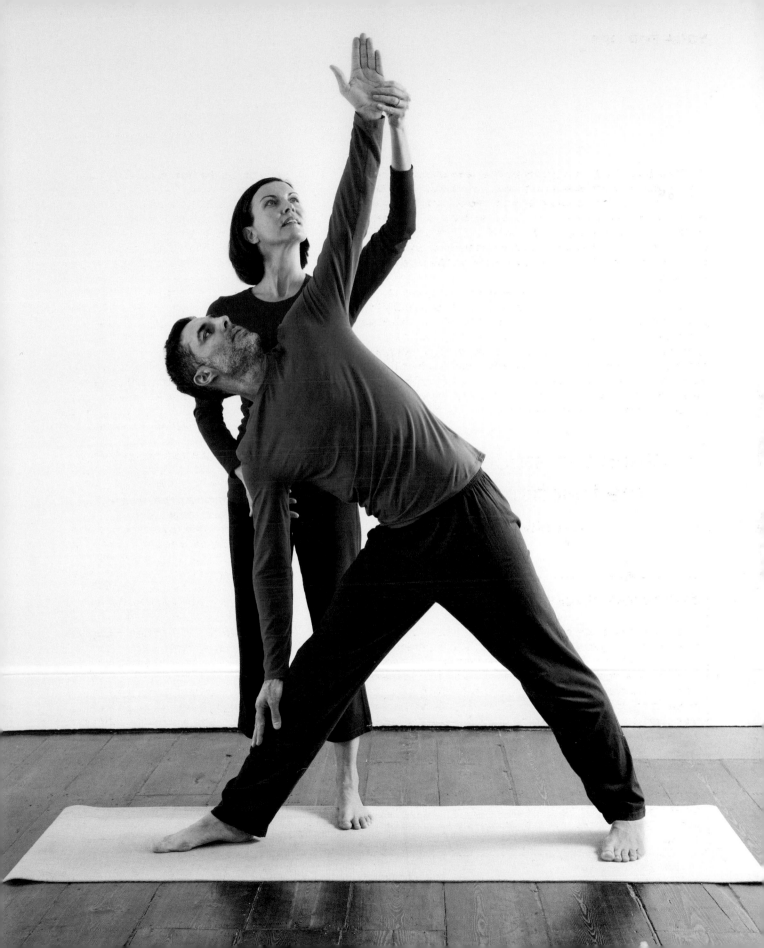

about most teacher-training programmes is available on search engines. Look up how long the teacher had to train for, and what kind of classes he or she is qualified to offer. Most reputable yoga centres have online biographies of their teachers, which make a good starting point – they also save you from having to ask the teacher personally, if that makes you feel uncomfortable.

Ask yourself if the setting's right I own and run a yoga studio in my home town, which is the distillation of everything I liked and enjoyed in other yoga studios I've visited over the years and around the world. It's light and airy. It's warm on a cold day (centrally-heated) and cool on a hot one (windows front and back, for a blissful seasidey through-breeze). It's uncluttered and features a few carefully chosen pieces of furniture and artwork: a Ganesh painting from Rajasthan, a Buddha head I've owned for years, a Balinese bench that students can sit on while they take off and put on their shoes, and a carved strip of Indian pegs. There's also a separate spacious loo (well, a couple) for changing, for students who prefer a little privacy. I created the studio this way because I've learned that the setting for yoga really can affect how much I want to go to a class.

When assessing your yoga space, ask yourself whether it feels calm. Is the ceiling high enough, or do you feel claustrophobic in the space? Is it freezing cold on a cold day? I had to stop going to a class in a local church hall, even though the teacher was fantastic, because it was heated by a single bar fire and the concrete floor made me feel as if I was in a cold storage facility. One of the most important factors to consider if you're less-than-happy changing in front of others is whether there is a place to get changed, or even – though this is a rare luxury – shower after class. By all means give any class a go, but if the venue doesn't feel inviting, you probably won't return that often.

This is the room that literally changed my life when I walked into a run-down ex-council buliding – and had the vision of how beautiful and inviting it could be, as a yoga studio

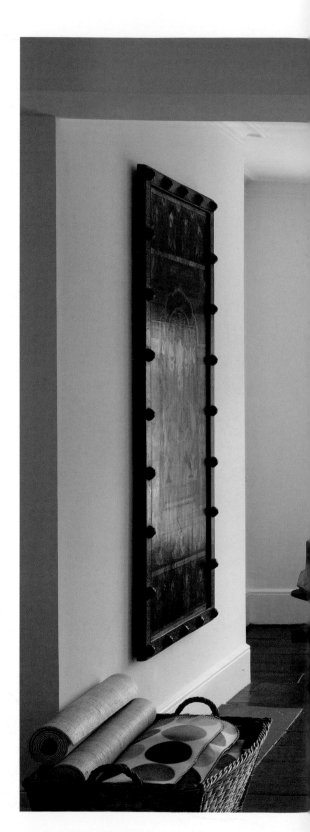

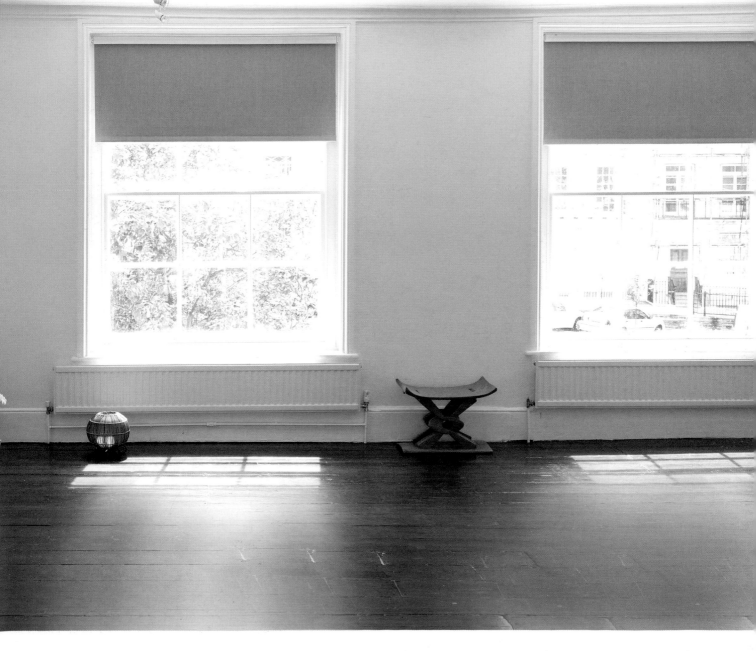

'Yoga is 99% practice and 1% theory'

Sri Krishna Pattabhi Jois (yoga guru)

BEST STYLES OF YOGA FOR OLDER BODIES

There is a reason why this book doesn't have a photograph of a fabulous older woman doing a headstand or a crab-like backbend on the cover. Or, for that matter, a shot of the famed yoga guru BKS Iyengar, who can contort himself like a pretzel at the age of ninety-something (at the time of writing).

That's because I believe that as we approach or reach mid-life, most of us are pretty realistic about what our bodies can achieve. The yoga books for older bodies on my bookshelf have generally been written by teachers who've practised yoga day in, day out for 30 years or so – and I think they give a more-than-slightly unrealistic picture not only of what can be achieved, but what most of us actually want from yoga. OK, if you were a veritable Olga Korbut as a teenager and have maintained your gymnastic flexibility ever since, that's one thing. But most of us creak a bit. We're happy to be able to touch our toes with ease and pick things up off the floor, without needing to hook our ankles behind our ears, Madonna-style. And I don't know about you, but I don't really want to be doing a major cardio-workout in class. If I want some aerobic exercise, I'm happy with a walk in the fresh air rather than trying to keep up with toned-tummied twenty-somethings in a hotbox studio. (Personally, I'd go out of my way to avoid any form of yoga that includes the word 'sweat' in the title.)

The postures – asanas, if you want to use the Sanskrit term – in this book are designed to improve flexibility, strength and resilience, but they're not going to get you a job in a circus anytime soon. If you're searching for a local yoga class, as well as knowing how to find your 'perfect' teacher (see pages 26–8), I think it's also important to have a run-down of the different styles of yoga, so you know what to expect.

DECIPHERING YOGA

With its impenetrable lexicon of Sanskrit words, slightly pedantic history and smattering of gurus with initials instead of names (such as BKS Iyengar or K. Pattabhi Jois), yoga can make you feel tied up in knots even before you go near a mat.

Top yoga teacher Simon Low acknowledges this, 'Yes, it is confusing. But these definitions aren't crucial. The teacher is far more important than the style. You'll know when you've found the right style for you, because every cell in your body will be saying "Yes!"'. Fundamentally, most styles of yoga embrace the same basic postures; what varies is the speed with which you 'transition' from one to another, how long the poses are held for, how often they're repeated – and how much of a spiritual element there is in a style or class. So on the following pages you'll find a basic 'yoga decoder' to help you decipher some of the most common styles of classes.

It's all about the teacher, and you may have to kiss a few frogs before finding your yogic prince or princess. When you do make that connection with the right person – when you just 'click' with a teacher – it can transform your experience, opening your eyes to aspects of yoga you've never thought about before

I've taken the bold step of giving a 'star rating' to the styles of yoga I think are most appropriate for the average person who hasn't done a lot of yoga but would like to start. This is subjective, based on what I've tried with my fifty-something body, and I've taken gazillions of different classes at different levels of challenge.

There are all sorts of wacky and/or new-new-new styles of yoga that I haven't even bothered to include here. In a marketing-driven world, individuals are always trying to put their 'stamp' on styles of yoga, to commercialise it. So you'll find 'hoop yoga' (hula hooping and yoga in a single class), 'acro yoga' (acrobatic yoga – making human pyramids!), 'Buddha camp' (a fusion of yoga and Pilates to a Bollywood techno soundtrack) and more. My advice? Stick to the basics until you've been doing this for a while. If you become obsessed and really want to explore and develop your yoga, then play around, but remember the golden rule: never, ever feel that you have to do anything, at any point, that's beyond your body's capabilities.

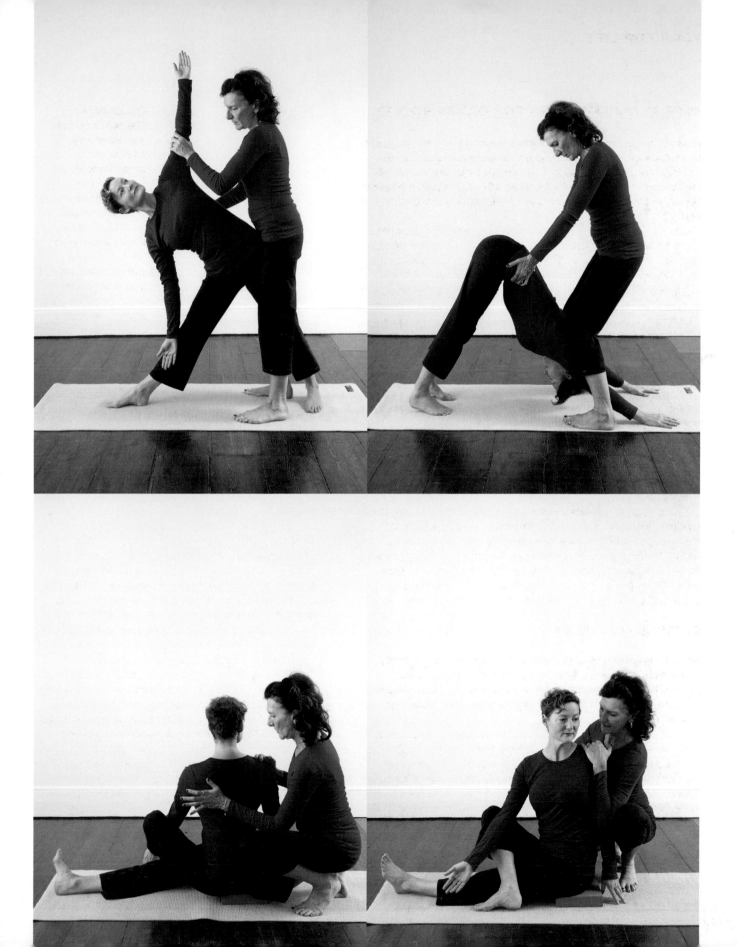

YOGA DECODER

ANUSARA**

Combines attention to alignment with awareness of the body's energy flow. This form of Hatha yoga (see below) has a very uplifting philosophy – 'a celebration of the heart' – and so most classes begin with a meditation and 'heart-orientated' sequence of flowing movements. Anusara is the Sanskrit word for 'flowing with grace'. Students of all levels of ability and yoga experience are generally welcome in Anusara classes.

ASTANGA*

Literally meaning 'eight limbs', Astanga is famously quite a fast-paced form. A specific set of poses is linked by swift flowing movements and synchronised with the breath. You start by learning a primary series, then progress to the secondary and finally an advanced series of postures, to create a flowing sequence of movement. It's physically demanding and challenging, involving jumping at times, and builds stamina and flexibility. Not for the faint-hearted, and (in my humble opinion), not really suitable for anyone taking up yoga in mid-life.

BIKRAM

OK, I haven't even given this style of yoga a star. That's because I just wouldn't recommend it for anyone who hasn't done a ton of yoga before. And if you're already having hot flushes, it's even less appropriate – because even if you're not menopausal, you'll get hot flushes in a Bikram class. Classes are based around a series of 26 energetic postures performed in high temperatures – around 40ºC/104ºF – designed to stretch muscles and expel toxins. This form takes its name from founder Bikram Choudhury, who sets very strict guidelines about what can and can't be taught in classes – which are, in my experience, very 'competitive'.

HATHA***

The style of yoga most widely taught in the West, using postures and breathing to discipline body and mind. The Sanskrit word hatha derives from ha (meaning 'sun') and tha ('moon'). It's the style that swept into the West with the first wave of hippies, but don't let that put you off. In my experience, most hatha yoga classes are an accessible mix of relatively gentle movements, maybe with some breathing exercises and a generous helping of relaxation at the end. Technically, all posture-based yoga should be labelled 'hatha', but the use of the word to advertise a class tends to mean something along the lines of what I've described.

IYENGAR***

Personally, I love Iyengar yoga and think it's very appropriate for mid-life and onwards. The focus in this form is on careful and precise alignment, and with a good Iyengar teacher you should develop an understanding of the 'living architecture' of the body. It is excellent for inner strength, stamina, flexibility, balance and concentration. BKS Iyengar, the founder of this form of yoga, often uses 'props' (such as blocks, belts and chairs) to help students experience postures, which I've found helpful. In Bridge Pose, for example, I was taught by an Iyengar teacher to put a block under the small of my back and relax onto that, which for my particular body type is fantastic for stretching out the area. Iyengar teachers are intensely schooled in anatomy and are particularly well equipped to train students to incorporate tiny adjustments into their practice, such as in toe and finger spacing, bringing openness and welcome stability to postures. Pick up any book on BKS Iyengar and marvel at the ninety-something guru himself, who's as bendy and sharp-witted as it's possible to be.

Star-rating key

* I wouldn't recommend this class for older bodies, unless you're already super-fit.
** OK, but a class I'd progress to, rather than start with.
*** Most likely to be doable/ enjoyable for older bodies.

'Yoga is a gift for older people. One who studies yoga in later years gains not only health and happiness but also freshness of mind, since yoga gives one a bright outlook on life. One can look forward to a satisfying, more healthful future rather than looking back into the past. With yoga, a new life begins, even if started later. Yoga is a rebirth which teaches one to face the rest of one's life happily, peacefully and courageously'

Geeta Iyengar

JIVAMUKTI*

The term Jivamukti literally means 'liberation while living'. This physically demanding and intellectually stimulating style of yoga rippled out from a famous New York studio of the same name, where each class has a spiritual theme and is supported by flowing sequences of postures, music and breathing exercises. It's hard work, although you usually get to rest at the end with some chanting and meditation.

KUNDALINI**

This style features all the classic hatha-yoga postures, but focuses on the controlled release of energy in the body, through the co-ordination of breath and movement, and meditation. There's a lot of focus on awakening energy (prana) at the foot of the spine and drawing it upwards through the chakras, energy centres situated along the spine, as well as on chanting and meditating on mantras such as Sat nam ('I am truth'). If you find this kind of talk annoyingly 'woo-woo', you may find that it gets in the way of enjoying the postures and breathing techniques.

POWER YOGA

No stars again. I'm afraid. This rebranding of Astanga yoga (see page 32), gives a good cardio (as well as muscle) workout, but is physically strenuous and demanding, making it less appropriate for relatively inexperienced and older bodies.

RESTORATIVE YOGA**

In the UK you're more likely to come across occasional Restorative yoga workshops than a regular class (more's the pity). Devoted to deep rest, these classes usually entail just a half-dozen or so poses held very passively with the support of bolsters, blankets and blocks. This makes it sound a bit like Yin yoga (see right), but I've found Restorative yoga slightly less stretchily demanding – although for beginners, it can be hard to hold poses for as long as is required, even with the proper supports. Possibly the most blissful part of this class is the ultra-deep relaxation at the end (20 minutes spent basically sinking into the ground), bringing true rest.

SCARAVELLI***

If you are lucky enough to have access to a Scaravelli class, run (or at least, gently jog) to sign up. This is a fantastic, non-aggressive style of yoga which (in my experience) is also hugely relaxing. Vanda Scaravelli – who developed this 'signature' style – was a Florentine Italian who studied yoga with BKS Iyengar (see previous page), but worked using gravity and the breath to help release tension in the body. The Scaravelli teachers I've experienced talk a lot about anatomy and posture, and in class you learn to make subtle postural adjustments – rather like in Pilates – that deepen the poses, which can be held for quite a long time. Because you're concentrating on alignment, this form is extremely relaxing – you simply don't have the brain-space to think about your to-do list or make holiday plans; you're right there on the mat. This approach is almost worthy of four stars, in my book – but alas, there aren't a huge number of Scaravelli teachers around, so it's a bit of a lottery as to whether you'll find one near you. Do book up for one-off workshops if you see them.

SIVANANDA**

I'd describe this (in not a terribly technical way) as a slightly souped-up version of Hatha yoga (see page 32) which emphasises 12 basic postures, repeated to build strength and flexibility of the spine. Classes are quite flowing (all the Sivananda teachers I've encountered have taught sun-salutation sequences), but there is also breath-work and sometimes chanting and meditation to help release stress and blocked energy. Some teachers focus on the physical side of Sivananda; others delve into the 'five fundamental points of yoga' as taught by Swami Sivananda, who founded the form: in addition to 'proper' exercise (the postures), there is 'proper breathing', 'proper relaxation' (Corpse Pose), 'proper diet' (vegetarianism) and positive thinking/meditation.

THERAPEUTIC YOGA***

Therapeutic yoga is a practice for those recovering from, or living with, illness or injury. Therapeutic yoga brings together supported poses, gentle yoga, breath-work and meditation – as well as hands-on healing, from some teachers – in a setting where your other classmates may be suffering from the same health challenges, such as lower back pain, or even cancer. These classes are not, as yet, terribly widely available, but if you do find one that seems to offer help with a challenge you're facing, do take extra time to talk through your situation with the teacher before a first class.

VINYASA FLOW YOGA**

This is a lovely fluid approach to yoga: vinyasa means linking movement to breath to create a smooth, fluid sequence. In other words: you don't get much rest-time between postures. Although this form is more 'forgiving' than Astanga, I wouldn't recommend it for total beginners; it's something to dip into to when you've built your strength and got your head around the postures, otherwise it's easy to be 'left behind' in sequences, which in turn can make you feel stressed.

YIN YOGA*

The roots of this style of yoga are said to be in the 'original' yoga, when ancient sages would sit for hours in contemplative meditation without moving. I absolutely love this type of yoga, in which you hold and surrender to deeply restorative (mostly) seated or reclining poses for long periods of time – from 3–5 minutes, or even as long as ten minutes in some classes. This is generally achieved with the help of 'props', such as bolsters, sandbags or perhaps an eye mask, and results in deep stretching of the connective tissues of the body (primarily around the hips, thighs and lower spinal area). I wouldn't recommend Yin yoga for novices: you can come out of some of these deep stretches feeling like a 90-year-old virtually fossilised in her armchair! But this form is definitely worth exploring once you are more experienced, since the postures do offer an astonishing stretch.

YOGA NIDRA***

Designed to help quiet over-active conscious minds, this form of yoga literally translates as 'yogic sleep', and basically guides you into a state of conscious deep sleep. You might seem to be asleep to an outsider – and yes, there is the risk when you begin these classes of that hideously embarrassing scenario of waking yourself by snoring – but being lulled into the deep state of mind between wakefulness and dreaming is tremendously relaxing and hugely restorative. For more details, see pages 160–4. Classes teaching this form are hard to find, but you might come across one-off workshops, or try a CD or download (see page 54).

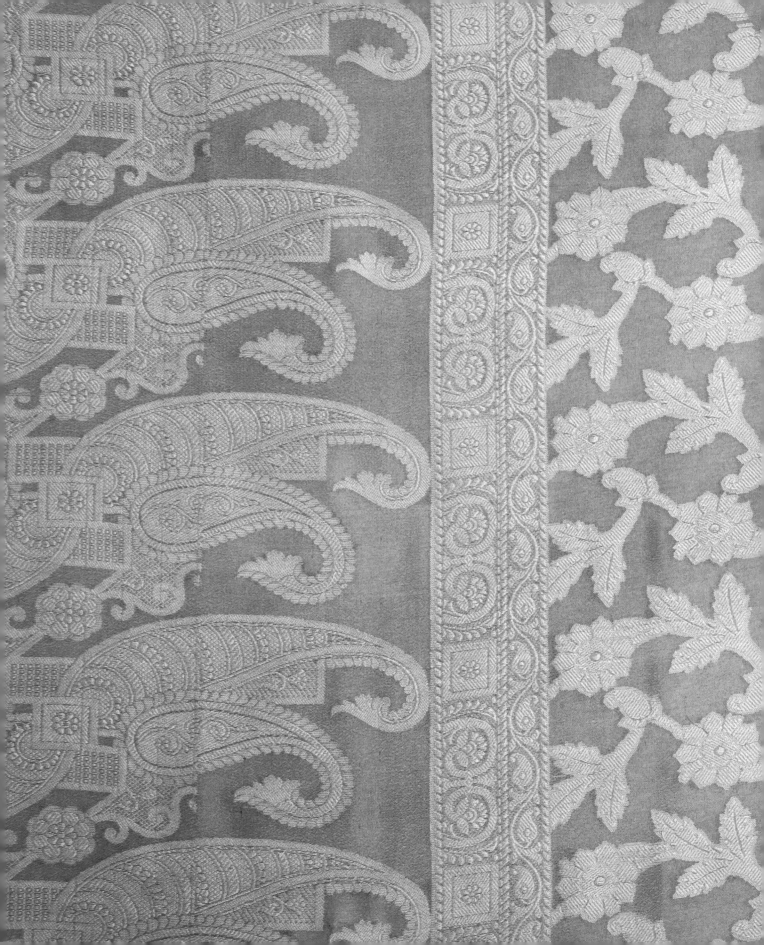

CHAPTER THREE

MAKING SURE 'OM' DOESN'T TURN INTO 'OUCH'

Like any form of physical activity, yoga can occasionally lead to injury – although according to American Sports Data, there are only two injuries per 10,000 yoga-practice sessions. In this book, aimed unashamedly at over-40s, I counsel you to avoid the very physically challenging types of yoga, which make it all too easy to push yourself too hard. Perhaps the other most useful piece of advice is to always 'listen' to your body. A very clever teacher once told me, 'There should always be two teachers in a class – the person leading the class, and your own body.'

The risk of injury in a class may actually be greater than during your home practice because – well, the human race is competitive by nature. No matter how often we're told 'Yoga isn't a competitive sport', it can be so tempting to sneak a sideways glance and compare your 'performance' with your neighbour's – and so push yourself that wee bit further into a forward bend, tugging dangerously on your hamstrings. I once found myself on an adjacent yoga mat to Ralph Fiennes in a Notting Hill yoga studio, and it took almost superhuman willpower not to push myself further than usual, to match his rather impressive bendiness. Likewise, it is folly mentally to compare yourself to, say, that famous photograph of Madonna with her leg hooked behind her ear. True yoga, as all the experts tell us, is about acceptance. Yes, you'll be keen to deepen your practice or improve your flexibility, that's only natural. But make the words 's-l-o-w-l-y' and 'g-r-a-d-u-a-l-l-y' your eternal watchwords. After all, the title of this book is *Yoga for Life* – nothing needs to happen overnight.

Happily, there are other practical ways to reduce your chances of becoming an injury statistic. Warming up properly is extremely helpful, of course, but you can further minimise your risk of injury by following this wisdom for a safe yoga practice:

TIP: SEE AN EXPERT

If you experience any severe or chronic (continuing or long-term) pain during your yoga practice, do see your doctor or consult a physiotherapist or chiropractor. This includes pain in the neck, shoulders and spine, numbness in your hands, and sharp pain in the wrists, fingers, elbows, shoulders or knees. I know many people with neck problems who have had excellent results from cranio-osteopathy, or craniosacral therapy, rather than the traditional 'bone-crunching' type of osteopathy. Your yoga teacher may be able to recommend a therapist. In general, a reputable therapist will offer free initial consultations.

AVOID 'KICK-BUTT' YOGA

Let's get real: 'fitness yoga' is generally inappropriate after your 30s. Quite often, this form of yoga is taught by exercise or aerobics teachers who've done little more than a bolt-on weekend course in yoga. At the risk of having a contract taken out on me by the owner of a chain of mirror-and-chrome gymnasiums, I advise you to avoid those sorts of yoga class like the plague.

SPEAK UP ABOUT INJURIES

Arrive early for a class if you haven't met the teacher before to introduce yourself and discreetly discuss any injuries or health issues past or present. This saves you from having to blurt out information about your hysterectomy/whiplash/hip operation in front of the whole class. Good teachers will always make suggestions for adaptations to postures to accommodate a bad knee, a dodgy back or a dicky hip. And if they don't? Only go as far as you're comfortable in a pose, and consider whether this is the teacher for you. (Refer back to my tips on finding the perfect teacher on pages 26–8.)

BE ON TIME

Running late for class can make injury more likely, especially if you miss warm-up sequences. Traffic problems, transport delays and last-minute calls do happen, but even if you're late into class, take a few breaths to ground yourself on your mat in Mountain Pose (see page 60) or Child Pose (see page 118) before joining in rather than being tempted to play catch-up or take a risky short-cut into a posture.

LISTEN TO YOUR BODY

Spend your first minute or two on the mat 'scanning' your body for existing aches and pains. Then subtly modify any poses that make them more painful, perhaps by using 'props' such as blocks or a belt. Better still, tell the teacher before the start of class (see above) about anything that's bothering you physically. A great teacher will introduce postures to the class that can

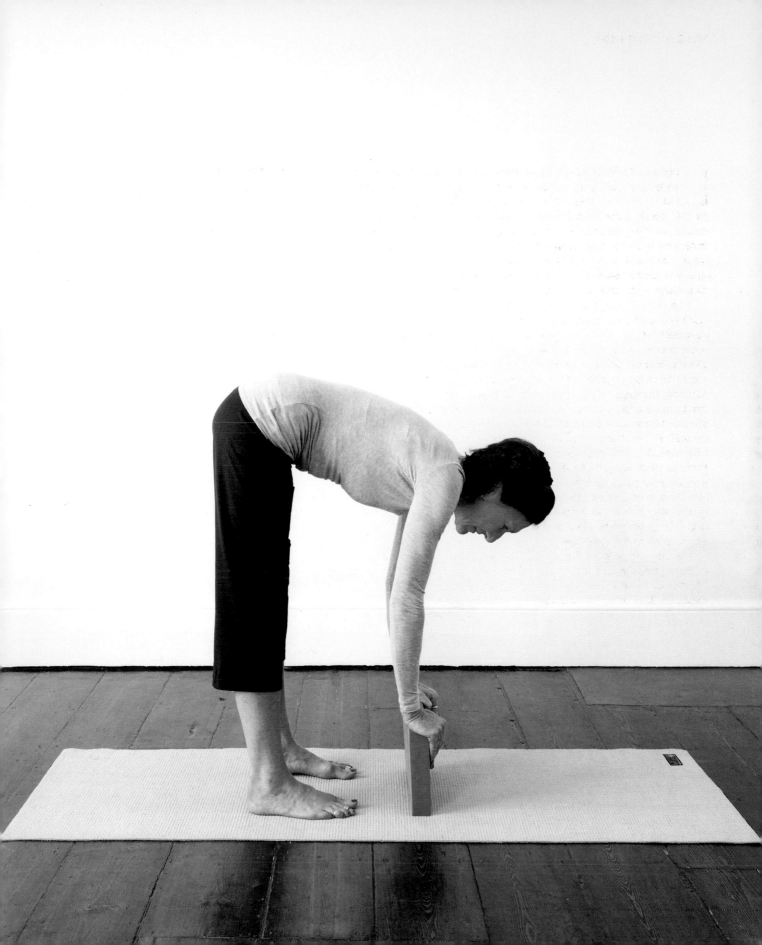

help, as well as helping you make adaptations to specific postures to suit your various niggles.

RESPECT YOUR 'EDGE'

At home or in class, listen to your body throughout your practice. Learn to feel the difference between 'good pain' (a great stretch), and 'bad pain' (anything that feels sharp). You should never push yourself that far, but if you do experience a jab of pain, don't work through it, thinking it will go away. This is likely to make it worse – instead, back off and rest, if you like. Child Pose (see page 118) is the default posture for resting and recovery, and it is absolutely OK to retreat into it at any time during your practice. If you continue to experience serious or chronic pain, see your doctor or a physiotherapist (see box on the preceding page).

HAVE THE RIGHT 'ATTITUDE'

Non-competitiveness is the spirit of yoga. To get used to this, think about checking in your ego with your shoes, by or outside the door. Try to start your practice with a feeling of surrender and acceptance, not impatience or angst.

DON'T FOLLOW THE HERD

Just because everyone else in the class can do something, that doesn't mean you have to. The reminder that yoga is non-competitive can't be repeated too often, especially if you've come to yoga later in life, when you may have to accept that you're not made of rubber like the twenty-something on the mat in front.

TUNE INTO DANGER SIGNALS

If your limbs start to shake when you're holding a posture, or you feel about to collapse, come out of a pose. Your strength will build gradually and one day you'll get there – but not now. Notice, too, whether you're having to open your mouth to breathe, or are breathing heavily – you may have gone past where you should be, so back off a bit, and perhaps rehydrate by taking a swig of water.

ALL DAYS ARE DIFFERENT

Bear in mind that you'll feel stronger on some days than others. This might be to do with how much sleep you've had (or haven't had), your diet, your general stress levels or emotional factors, or just biorhythms, if you believe in them. Some people, for example, find that they breeze through balances during a morning class, but can't stay upright in the same poses in the evening.

QUESTION SHOULDERSTAND

According to many experts, this is the yoga posture most likely to cause injuries in people over 40. I would certainly advise any yoga beginner to avoid Shoulderstand (let alone Headstand). I find it makes me deeply uncomfortable, stressed and breathless, and I agree with Dr. Stuart Kahn, of the Spine Institute of New York at Beth Israel Medical Centre, who says, 'Avoid headstands and shoulderstands until you have spent several years building the flexibility to perform them. When you do them, be extra careful when rolling up into position, as that's the most stressful part.' He also advises against dropping your legs over your head into what's known as Plough Pose (Halasana). Shoulderstand should also be avoided by anyone who is more than 13 kilos (around 29 pounds) overweight, since the additional weight places pressure on the neck and/or elbows. In this book you will find just one Shoulderstand – Supported Shoulderstand (see page 116) – which uses the support of blankets and a wall. Even then, build up to it up over a lengthy period of time. Alternatively, try the more comfortable inversion Legs-up-the-wall Pose (see page 114), which offers many of the benefits without the risks. If you're in the middle of a studio with no access to a wall, simply lie on your back and lift your legs at 90 degrees to your body, resting your hands, palms down, on either side of your body. You're not being wimpy; you're being savvy.

LOVE YOUR KNEES

Yoga is brilliant for strengthening the leg muscles – and when your quadriceps (those whacking great muscles at the front of the thigh) are strong, they take a lot of pressure off your knees. However, there are certain postures in which you need to take extra care of your knees, including Lotus Pose (Padmasana), Pigeon Pose (see page 96) and even Child Pose (see page 118). If knees are your problem zone, avoid moves that bend or twist the joint past your comfort point. Never force your legs into Lotus Pose; be content to sit cross-legged. And if you can't manage to sit cross-legged comfortably on the floor, lift your behind onto a bolster or block, which creates extra 'room' for your crossed legs.

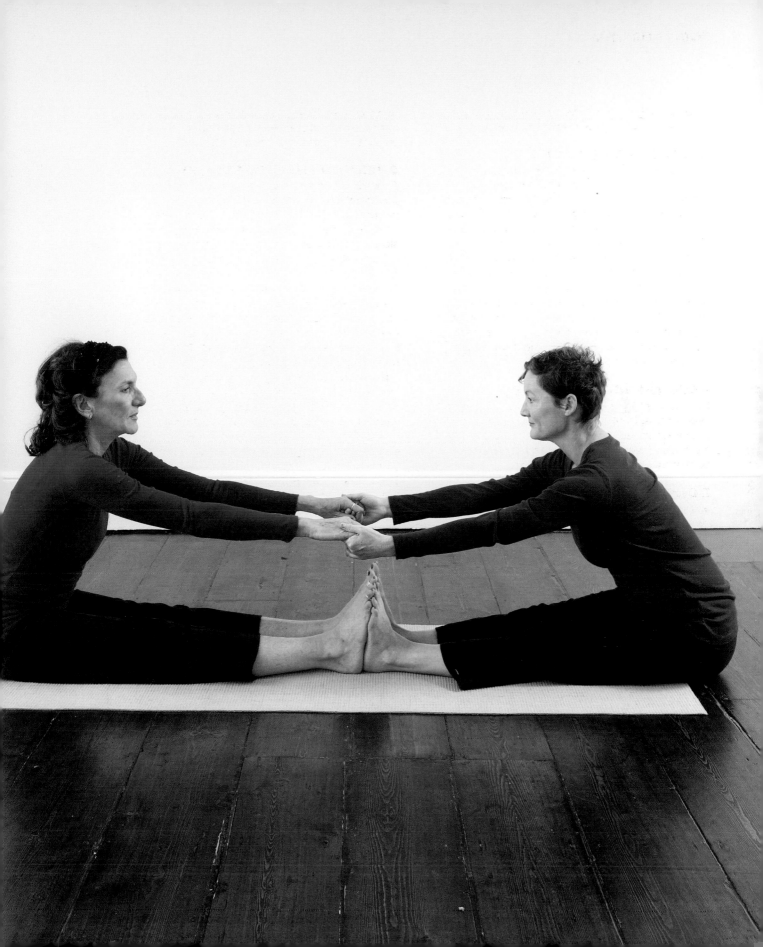

If you have injuries, ask your teacher for adjustments that will make poses safer. I can't do a traditional Child Pose because of two old injuries: a snapped Anterior Cruciate Ligament (ACL) in my right knee, and whiplash that affected the bottom of my neck. So instead of keeping my legs together, I place my knees much wider apart. And instead of resting my head on the ground, which puts pressure on my neck, I cushion my forehead with my hands.

AVOID DOWNWARD DOGITIS
Postures that put pressure on the wrists – such as plank-style poses, Upward-facing Dog Pose (see page 98) or Downward-facing Dog Pose (see page 64) – can feel very stressful. We're simply not used to putting weight on our hands – and time spent typing at computers also affects our wrists, which have to make thousands of repetitive movements we just didn't evolve to execute. While you are building your strength and stamina, limit the amount of time you spend on your hands. It can also help to 'cushion' the wrists, either by folding your yoga mat back on itself, creating an extra layer of sponginess beneath the wrists, or by using a 'squishy' foam block.

WHEN YOU ARE IN POSTURES
that put weight on your hands, be sure to draw your shoulderblades back and down. If your arms and shoulders are weak, strengthen them by practising very gentle lifts and bicep curls at home, using regular cans of food, such as baked beans, as weights. (Much cheaper than a special set of weights!) If you ever feel numbness in your hands or sharp pain in your wrists, fingers, elbow or shoulders, it's time to seek help from your doctor or a physiotherapist.

FOLLOW SOME BACK BASICS
Do some general mobility exercises, such as shoulder rolls (see photos opposite) and light stretching before you start a yoga class. A little T'ai Chi-style 'swaying' (see page 123) can also help to warm up your spine. The stronger your abdominal muscles, the more they'll help to stabilise your back, so think about practising a few gentle sit-ups at home, too. In general, yoga

Doing some general mobility exercises such as shoulder rolls is a great way to warm up before a yoga class

is fantastic for stomach-strengthening – that famous 'yoga tummy' – even if those toned muscles are buried under a little excess avoirdupois after a certain age. If you have issues with your lower back, though, do take it very easy in twisting and forward bending poses.

ADJUSTMENTS
Sometimes in a class, a yoga teacher will move around the room adjusting students's alignment, or even using their body weight to push them deeper into a pose. If you've already reached your limit, say so. Don't feel that you have to go a fraction of a millimetre deeper into a posture than is totally comfortable. For instance, because of my ancient (skiing-related) knee injury, I understand I can't get as deeply into Child Pose (see page 118) as I'd like. So I always quietly tell a teacher who's just put her hand on my neighbour's back to encourage her to sink further into Child that I'm fine as I am, thanks. A good teacher will respect individual difference rather than force everyone to get their palms on the floor in forward bends and kick up into headstands.

MAKE A RECORDING
I taught myself yoga using a book, so I absolutely know it can be done – but I also know that trying to keep one eye on the page while you get into a posture can be awkward and strain the body. So if you have a voice recorder on your smartphone or a digital tape recorder, try making a recording of the instructions for the sequences of postures on page 123. Then, for a safe practice, just play the recording back and follow the instructions. Be sure to read slowly when you are recording, and leave enough pauses so that you can rest in postures for the allotted time. This tip requires a bit of preparation, but I have found that listening to my own commands is just about the only way I can successfully practice yoga at home. I can focus better on the instructions and screen out the invariable distractions of my home environment (looking at fluffballs under the bed, thinking about the work day ahead, or what I've got to prepare for supper etc).

'Yoga calms me down. It's a therapy
session, a workout and meditation,
all at the same time'

Jennifer Aniston

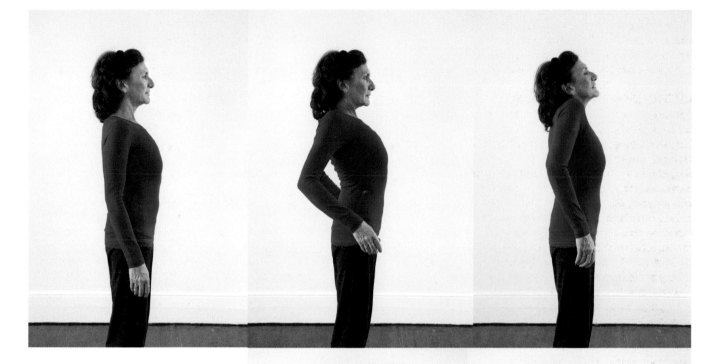

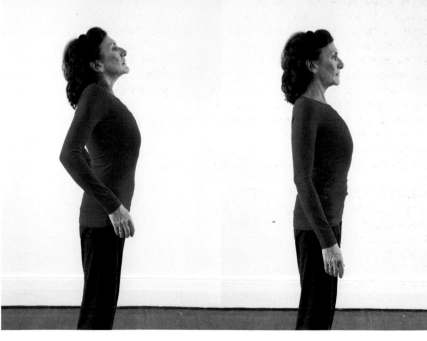

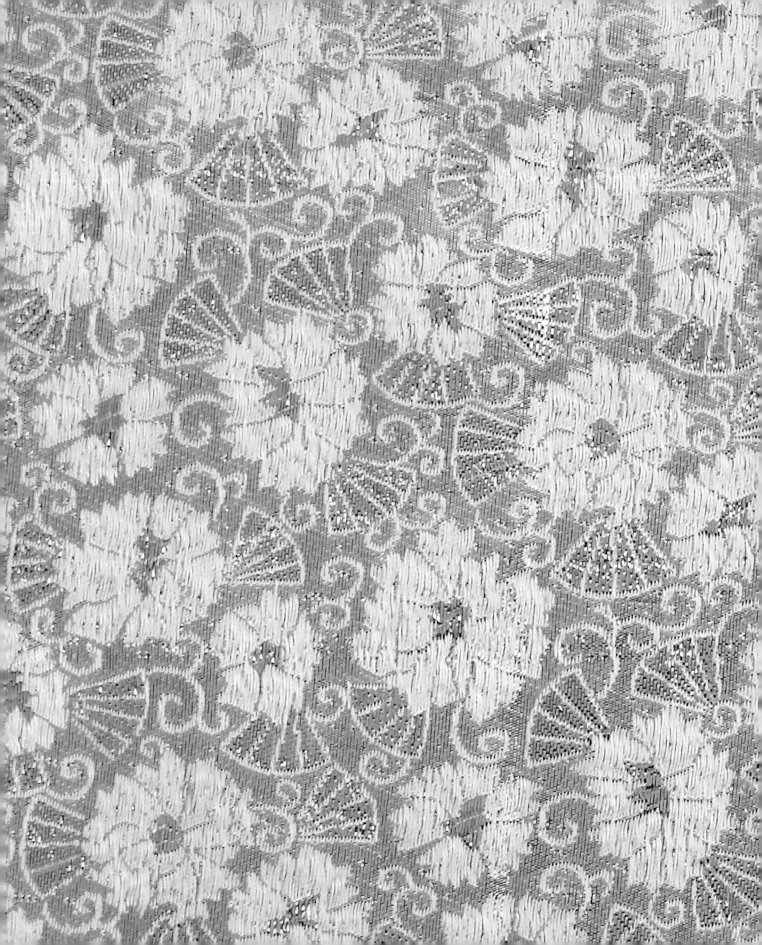

CHAPTER FOUR

YOUR YOGA SPACE
AT HOME

Wherever I lay my mat (that's my home)… to paraphrase Marvin Gaye. And it's true: all you really need for a great home yoga practice is a sticky mat and enough space around it to extend 360 degrees into the poses. The reality is, though, that it takes discipline to make yourself practise at home, and not be distracted by the urge to check e-mails, put on another load of laundry or check the messages on your phone.

So carving out a dedicated space for your home practice really, really helps – if you can manage it. It doesn't have to cost much; after all, you're doing this to express yourself, not to impress another soul. And it doesn't require a whole room; a corner of a room is fine. But if you can't dedicate a whole room to your practice, at least try to block off your yoga space with a beautiful screen. Wherever your special yoga space is, you will find that it becomes a refuge and an oasis – and so your mind automatically starts to relax whenever you get on the mat. Here are my tips on creating the perfect space at home.

'The word yoga comes from Sanskrit, the language of ancient India. It means union, integration, or wholeness. It is an approach to health that promotes the harmonious collaboration of the human being's three components: body, mind, and spirit'

Stella Weller (yoga author)

CHOOSE A HARD FLOOR

You'll be practising yoga on a mat, of course, but a rubber mat plus a squishy carpet is tougher for balancing poses. There is also something wonderfully grounding about practising yoga on wood or stone (or bamboo, a fantastic new eco-friendly flooring material). On the other hand, if you're worried about falling, practising on carpet can make you feel safer. If you have a very hard floor (say, slate), you may need a thicker yoga mat (look for those intended for Astanga practice), or you might like to try doubling up with one mat on top of another, which can be gentler on the joints.

BANISH THE CLUTTER

To create a sense of peace, you might not want to go as far as creating an altar or buying yourself a statue of the Hindu god Ganesh. But do make sure your yoga space is clear of clutter. Move old photograph albums, dusty tennis rackets or piles of paperwork – they will only distract you from your practice. Keep the walls unadorned or go for simple, uncomplicated images. Patterned wallpaper and strong colours can also be a distraction; there's a reason most yoga studios are painted in calming creams and neutrals (with maybe a touch of earthy red or brown) – it works. A mirror, meanwhile, is entirely optional. It can be good for checking your alignment, but if you'd really rather not look at yourself while practising, I empathise entirely.

GET THE LIGHTING RIGHT

Natural light is perfect for practising yoga, but if the only place you can carve out enough room for your little yoga corner is a dark attic, go for it. While sunlight is energising, direct sun can make you feel hot (or even, yes, flushed). If your space gets lots of direct sun, consider fixing

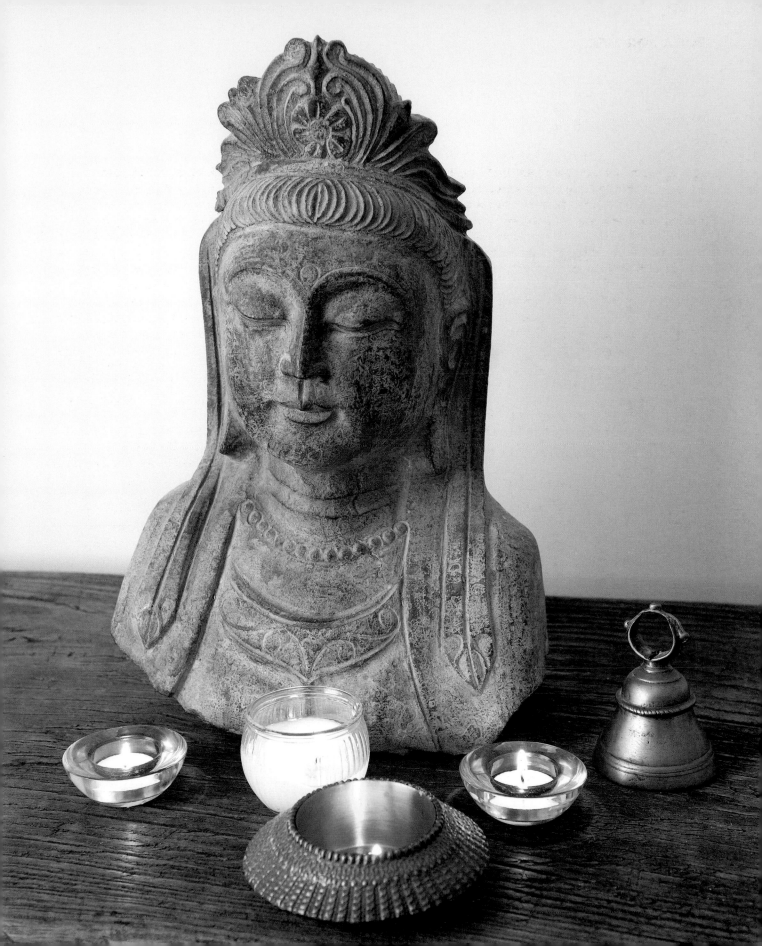

up a lightweight blind or soft sheeting – unless you have a view of the garden or countryside and like to be inspired by changing seasons. (Me? I'd find it hard not to get out there and start weeding, and so would prefer the blind.) In windowless spaces or for after-dark practice, opt for soft, shaded lighting; lying on the floor with a halogen bulb blasting your retinas does not feel very yogic. Candles are great, but the usual warnings about leaving them unattended or placing them too close to soft furnishings apply (no less than three of my friends have managed to create small house fires with candles).

THINK ABOUT MUSIC

On page 54 you'll find a list of terrific yoga soundtracks, but you might find that playing birdsong, Eastern-influenced music or Western classical music makes your yoga practice more focused. Maybe you prefer the sound of silence – some people find music distracting. You'll only find out what makes your yoga space most conducive to regular practice by experimenting. If you need a CD player or iPod speakers to play music, try and position them well away from your workout area so they don't constrain any of your movements or (sorry to sound like a naggy health-and-safety officer) become a trip hazard.

MAKE SURE IT'S WARM ENOUGH

The temperature of your home yoga space should be warm enough that you feel comfortable sitting still in a t-shirt and yoga pants. Keep a blanket to hand to cover yourself during a long final relaxation or meditation session. If your yoga space is cold and draughty, you won't practice; it's as simple as that. On the other hand, on a hot day (or during hot flushes), it's fantastic to be able to open a window or turn on a fan for a cooling breeze.

Carving out a dedicated home yoga space to practice in really, really helps. It doesn't require a whole room; a corner of a room or small area that you can screen off from the rest of the room is fine

SANCTIFY YOUR SPACE

If you do want to make an altar in your yoga space, don't feel like a weirdo. Plenty of people do. It doesn't mean that you've changed your religion (or even found one); an altar can simply give you something to focus on or anchor you when you're meditating. (For more details, see pages 140–1.) To make an altar, use any small table or cut down a console table and paint it or throw a cloth over it. Place whatever feels calming on your altar table: nature photos, fresh flowers, statues of deities, a bell, candles. I have a small painted Indian altar that I found cheaply in a junk shop, and on it I keep a few objects that mean something to me. The most significant is my small brass bell. Nothing stills my mind like the lingering vibration of a bell, and I have 'auditioned' hundreds of bells in my time to find the 'perfect' sound, remembering what a local antique dealer once said to me: that a bell should have 'the cry of a child' in its ring. Aside from this single piece of furniture, it can be wonderful to keep your home yoga space furniture-free.

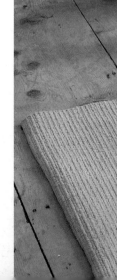

'A lot of exercise is mindless;
you can have music or the radio on and not be aware.
But if you're aware in anything you do -
and it doesn't have to be yoga - it changes you.
Being present changes you'

Mariel Hemingway

YOUR YOGA KIT

In India, all a yogi needs is a square metre of earth and something to focus on. Personally, I'm all for a bit of yoga 'kit' – not as some kind of fashion statement or status symbol, but because it can actually make practising easier.

Yoga has of course become big business – no, huge business – with countless 'shopportunities' designed, I guess, to make us feel a little more 'yogic'. Being something of an inveterate shopper, I've done quite a bit of expensive personal research into what's worth the money, and what's non-essential. Quite a lot of this, if I need to justify myself, was while I was setting up my own yoga studio, when I really needed to know which were the best mats, belts, bolsters and so on. So here's the best of what's out there, with tried and tested suggestions for what you need and what you don't. For details of where to find the best products online, see pages 220–21.

THE WHAT-TO-WEAR DILEMMA

It is, of course, perfectly possible to do yoga in a scruffy old t-shirt and a pair of shorts or leggings. The most important thing is to be comfortable, and frankly not to give a damn what anyone else thinks about your choice of yoga gear. However, when it comes to yoga pants, I would recommend finding some with a bit of 'give', and preferably with a wide elastic panel around the waist. You don't want to be hitching your 'bottoms' up while you're getting into postures, nor do you want to feel as if your tummy's rolling out over the elastic – or bulging, muffin-top-style, come to that.

The best yoga pants When you don't have a flat stomach, some yoga pants roll down and need constant hitching up – a serious distraction. Many yoga pants on the market have a low waistline and sit on the hips, which may not be terribly comfortable either. Of all the yoga pants I've tried and recommended to friends, Gossypium's Cropped Foldover Trouser (see page 220)

is a universal hit. There's a bit of Lycra in the super-wide foldover waistband which keeps your tummy in place (and your trousers in place, at the same time). These come to mid-calf (I'm 5' 5"), and are also available as a Long Foldover Trouser, if you prefer something that reaches your ankles. Though I would say that it's very important to see all of your feet, in yoga, to be able to make adjustments, which is why I prefer cropped pants. PrAna, who also make terrific sustainable yoga-wear, offer a similar style in each new collection (see page 220). If you can't get hold of these brands, look for any yoga pants with a wide, foldover waistband – they truly do stay up and give a wobbly abdomen a bit of support.

If you have great legs and are happy to show them off, then by all means wear leggings for your practice. But in my experience these can make you feel a bit hot, and if you aren't 100 per cent happy with your legs, whether you feel they're too skinny or on the curvaceous side, you may feel a bit self-conscious in class.

For men, knee-length jersey shorts seem to be the way to go – or try longer yoga pants. You may at times want to roll up the leg of your pants – for instance, for Tree Pose (see page 70) – so tracksuit bottoms with their elasticated ankles aren't ideal.

The top tops I personally like a v-necked t-shirt (it lets my neck and chest 'breathe' when I get hot in class). However, in inverted postures, baggy t-shirts can end up around your armpits, exposing your tummy and chest to one and all. (Be sure to tuck a loose top in before heading upside down.) Again, it's up to you how much flesh you like to expose in a yoga class; there are many body-conscious yoga tops or vests out there with a percentage of elastane for fit. These allow you to move into a pose without restriction, but if you aren't happy (yet) with your body, they can make you feel a bit bulgey. Again, you may want to check out the prAna range for yoga tops (see page 220). Gossypium (see page 220)

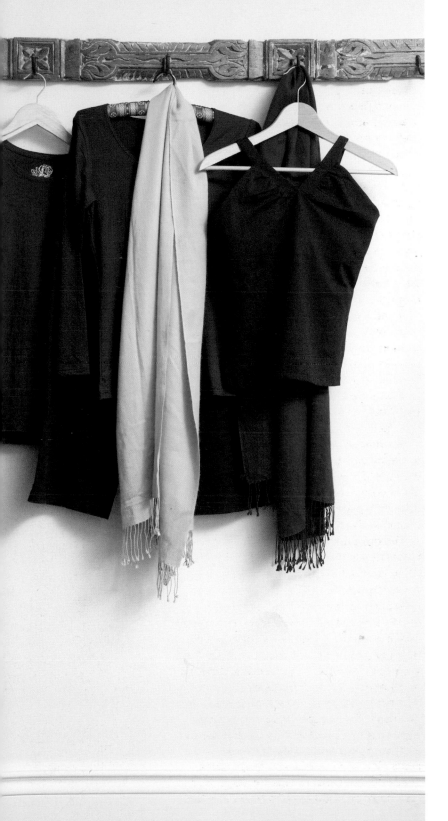

also offers a stretch 'dress' that covers the hip and upper thigh area in a forgiving way, and has just the right amount of 'give' to let you ease into even the bendiest pose.

FINDING THE PERFECT MAT You don't absolutely need your own mat if you're going to a class, since most yoga centres keep a stash of mats. The downside? These communal mats can become a bit 'whiffy' if they're not cleaned regularly. (I am somewhat Howard Hughes-like about ensuring the mats at my own yoga centre are washed thoroughly and often.) Layering your own mat on top of the mat that's been provided can offer extra cushioning and a familiar feel, which can be welcome in a class setting.

I have tried loads and loads of mats and my absolute favourite is the prAna mat (see page 220). It's slightly more expensive than most, but it is expensive for good reason – it offers great 'grip' and is springy without being over-springy – and is a favourite of many yoga teachers, for its durability and performance. I've found that some thick mats are too 'bouncy', and can make it harder to find and keep your balance. The materials in the prAna mat are non-toxic and biodegradable; it's PVC-free and comes in cool colours. I have given these mats to yoga-loving friends who are all fans. prAna also make a very lightweight travel yoga mat that folds without getting creased.

I am also a fan of the Ecoyoga mat (see page 220), which is based on latex and jute fibres and is nicely non-slip (this is the one I chose when equipping my own yoga studio). Again, this is not the cheapest yoga-mat choice out there, but it is very durable. Importantly, neither of these two mats smell very synthetic. For me, this is a real issue – if I am spending a lot of time with my nose up-close-and-personal with a yoga mat, I don't want toxic 'fumes' in my face.

KEEP IT CLEAN Yoga mats should be cleaned regularly. Wipe your own mat down with a towel after use, and/or spritz it with the Yoga Mat Spray mixture below, to leave it smelling clean. Roll it up after the surface has dried. For light marks and dirt, add a few drops of dishwashing liquid to 500ml water, then, using a damp, non-scratchy cleaning sponge or a towelling rag, clean the mat, rubbing any soiled areas with the soapy water. Wipe the mat with a clean, wet cloth, making sure you remove all the soap – any residue can cause slipperiness. Dry your mat with a towel before hanging it to dry completely over a washing line or airer (don't hang it over a heated towel rail unless you want a permanent 'kink' in the mat).

YOGA MAT SPRAY Essential oil of tea tree and lavender have natural antimicrobial and antibacterial properties and a history of use in cleansing – as well as a wonderfully refreshing scent. They form the basis of this mat spray. If you don't have these staple oils in a home remedy kit, you can buy them relatively inexpensively online, or substitute peppermint oil, which also has an energising and uplifting scent. You will need a clean bottle with a pump-action spray top to store the spray.

> **240ml water**
> **60ml witch hazel**
> **60 drops essential oil (choose from lavender, tea tree or peppermint)**

Place all the ingredients in the bottle, screw on the top and shake everything together well. To use, shake well, then spray onto the mat from a close distance – 5cm or so – and use a towel or a piece of paper towel to wipe the mat down. Allow to dry completely before rolling up the mat.

PROP YOURSELF UP For a home-yoga practice I have found the following 'props' make it easier to get into, remain in or relax into poses.

BRICKS AND BLOCKS A rectangular-shaped brick is very useful for supporting your hand in Triangle Pose (see page 68). I recommend cork, which is more sturdy than foam bricks. Blocks are thinner and wider than bricks. I recommend two hard foam blocks, plus a half-block. Use the hard blocks to keep you symmetrical in poses, for support when you can't reach as far to the ground as you'd like. The half block is useful when placed beneath your head during final relaxation, or use it to cushion wrists that feel pressured in certain poses. Lightweight foam is best for the full-size blocks, 'squishy' soft foam for the half-thickness block. A 'wedge' can be helpful if you find it hard to get your heels to the ground when you're squatting, or you'd like a little extra support beneath your heels in Downward-facing Dog Pose (see page 64). These are available in foam, but some yogis prefer wood or cork.

BOLSTERS AND BLANKETS These are invaluable, if for nothing else then relaxation: place a bolster or folded thick woollen blanket beneath your knees to elevate them, and then lie flat on your back. If you have any back-health 'issues', it can be much more comfortable to elevate the knees on a bolster during final relaxation. Round bolsters are used widely, but you can also find oblong bolsters which can be useful for supporting knees or hips in seated poses. At home, you can use firm cushions instead. When choosing blankets to support the body, good old-fashioned wool blankets are best, rather than fleecy or squishy blankets. The clue is in the word 'support'!

BELTS OR STRAPS To extend your reach, loop a strap around your foot when stretching out your legs, or grasp the ends between your hands if they don't meet in a pose. Choose one with a D-ring, which won't slip, but allows you to adjust the length easily when you're in a pose. Belts come in different widths – experiment in a class to find which you prefer. At home you could substitute a scarf.

BAGS In some poses it can feel comforting to have a sandbag (like those used in schools) resting on part of your body to promote relaxation; sandbags can also be used to encourage parts of the body, such as the thighs, to relax into a stretch. Eye bags or pillows filled with flax seeds can be lovely to help you relax in the final moments of a yoga session, and there are instructions for making and using one on page 124.

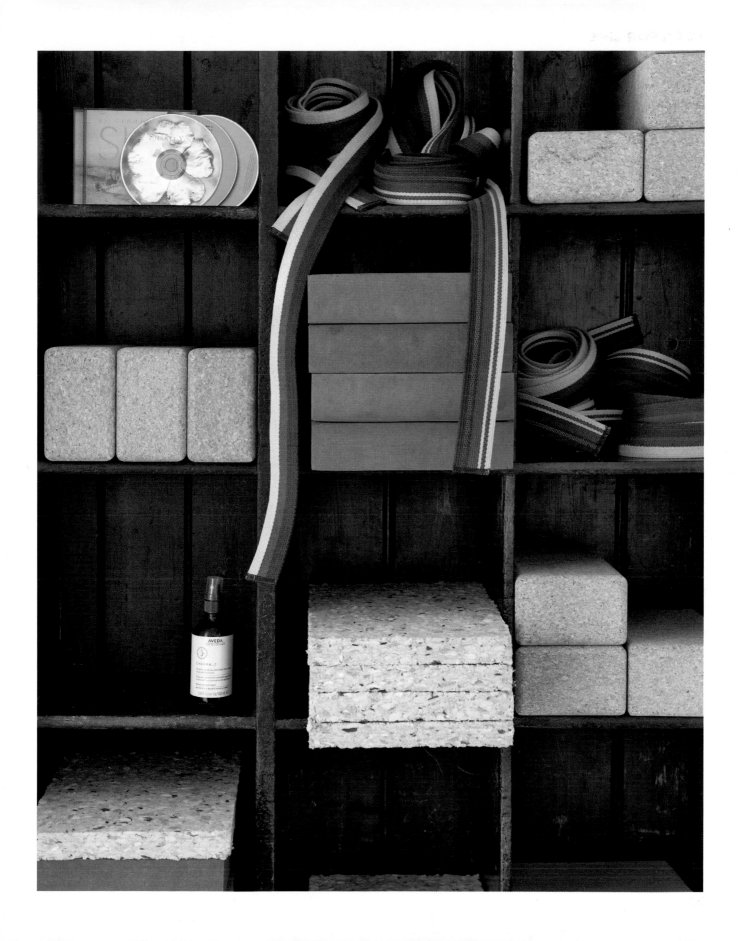

LITTLE EXTRAS The following suggestions are not essential, but make any yoga space feel a little more inviting.

PASHMINA OR SHAWL This is to drape over you in relaxation. You might prefer a fleece fabric to wool or silk. I used to be a bit of a purist, thinking that synthetic fabrics had no place in a 'natural' environment like a yoga studio. Until, that is, I was seduced by some 'snuggle touch' fleece blankets (see page 220), which are super-warm and ultra-light as well as being incredibly soft to the touch and just fantastic for relaxation.

INCENSE Some people love incense in class; others find it brings on a coughing fit, especially if used during asana work rather than simply before the class begins. If you like incense, check out the Himalaya Spa Incense range (see page 220), which uses the highest quality essential oils (unlike cheap Indian incense, which is often synthetically fragranced). It comes in does-what-it-says-on-the-packet varieties which include Clear Thoughts, Happy Heart, Meditation, Pure Air, Sweet Dreams and Quiet Mind.

WHAT YOU DON'T NEED There are a lot of yoga gear manufacturers out there, seeking to get their hands on your cash. I am not sure anyone needs toe separators, for instance. A regular yoga practice will help your feet to spread naturally – which is good for the health of your feet and for overall balance, and is a real bonus if your toes have been crammed into tight shoes for years. There are many, many other yoga 'accessories' that you can shop for: head-bands, sweat-bands, super deluxe mats (I recently saw one for £180 with 'jewel' detail!), pricey yoga mat sprays and sexily-embroidered carrying bags. As long as you've got a mat, and something comfy to wear, you're basically sorted.

MUSIC If you find background sounds enhance your practice, you will need a CD player or iPod speakers, Of course, you can practise yoga while listening to just about any music you like as well as in silence. If your yoga teacher plays music you like, ask for his or her recommendations. Having listened to many, many yoga CDs and downloads, here is my personal playlist. I like deep, grounding sounds rather than whale song, and I also find that crystal bowl and 'singing bowl' sounds are fantastic for meditation. All the following can be accessed through iTunes so you can listen before you buy.

Here are some of my favourite albums for yoga and relaxation.

YOGA PLAYLIST
108 Sacred Names of Mother Divine: Sacred Chants of Devi – Craig Pruess and Ananda
All One – Krishna Das
Domain of Shiva – Sat-Kartar Kaur
Door of Faith – Krishna Das
Gathering in the Light – Baird Hersey and Prana with Krishna Das
Kamasutra Experience – Al Gromer Khan
Music for Deep Meditation
Tibetan Singing Bowl – David Harshada Wagner
Music for Yoga and Other Joys – Jai Uttal
Mystic India 2 (compilation; various artists)
Prana Yoga (compilation; various artists)
Quiet Mind: The Musical Journey of a Tibetan Nomad – Nawang Khechog
Satori: Music for Yoga and Meditation – Riley Lee and Gabriel Lee
Sufi – Al Gromer Khan
Sundari and *Music for Slow Flow Yoga I and II* – Gabrielle Roth (also pretty much anything by Gabrielle Roth)
Tantra Drums – Al Gromer Khan
The Oneness Mantra – Ananda Giri
Tibetan Bowl Meditations – River Guerguerian
Yoga Mela (compilation; various artists)
Yoga: On Sacred Ground – Chinmaya Dunster
Yoga Spirit – Akasha

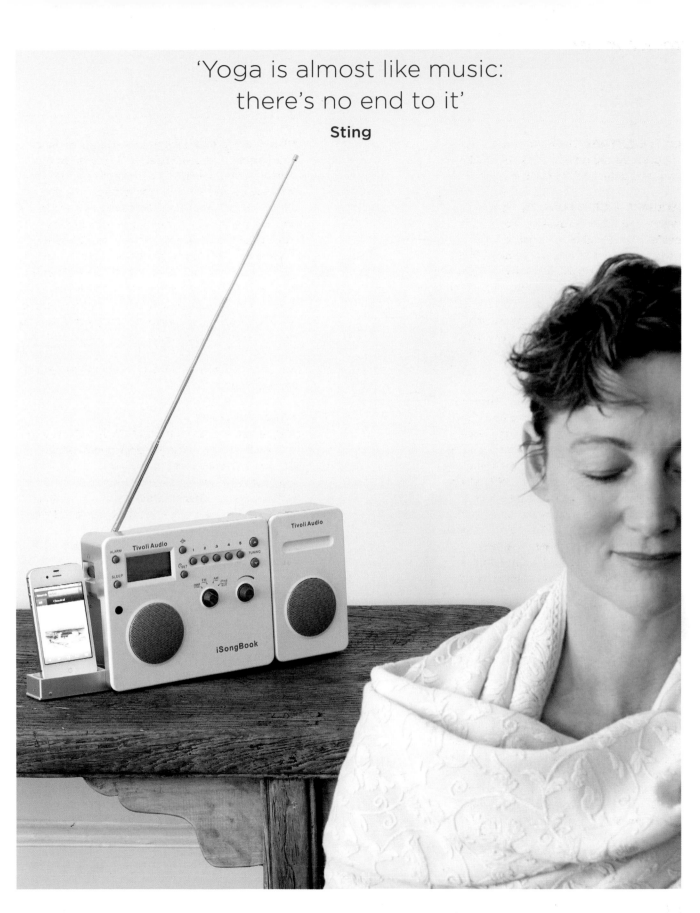

'Yoga is almost like music:
there's no end to it'
Sting

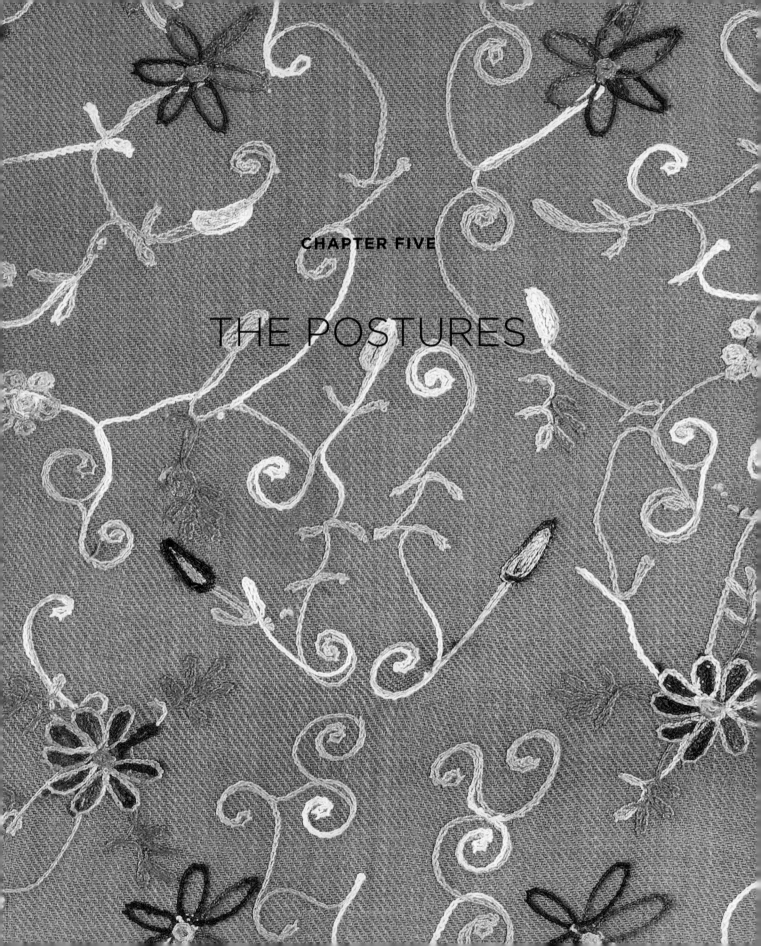

CHAPTER FIVE

THE POSTURES

On the following pages you'll find instructions for many yoga postures – asanas, to give them the Sanskrit name – which should be achievable for those who are new to yoga, at any age and all stages of life. Is this selection of poses totally comprehensive? Nope. You won't find headstands or handstands, postures that are likely to strain a back that's unfamiliar with arching strongly, or poses that might put excessive pressure on a fragile knee.

What you will find is a range of poses that you can do at home and which will give your body all the workout it truly needs. To quote yoga teacher Tom Briggs, who founded Turtle Island Yoga in San Rafael, California, 'I don't see the need to do the really "fancy" poses – the ones at the back of the book, so to speak. I find the same benefit in the simpler poses.' I quite agree, which is why this book is the way it is. And if you do want to take things further, turn to the booklist on page 221.

BEFORE YOU START

Before you take to the mat, read over these few simple guidelines to ensure that your yoga practice is both effective and safe. Then follow the step-by-step instructions very carefully, not only to avoid injury but to get maximum benefits. The golden rule is to ease into and out of postures slowly and with intention, and to breathe properly throughout.

Practise regularly But how often is enough? In a perfect world, you would do at least 30 minutes of yoga practice three times a week. In an imperfect world (the one we live in), just practise as often as you can manage, for as long as you can manage. I find there's a certain 'magic' to yoga: if I take time out of a busy schedule for my practice, I feel like I have more time. To begin with, don't be over-zealous about practising; build up the time you spend on the mat gradually and slowly. But do try to keep the practise regular, not least because family and friends are more likely to respect that time you're taking and not try to intrude. Regularity is the key to seeing and experiencing the benefits of yoga. That said, something is always better than nothing. Even stepping away from your desk for a Downward-facing Dog (see page 64) is better than just sitting there.

Figure out your 'best time' for yoga There are no hard and fast rules for this. I'll leave the advice to renowned yoga teacher Cyndi Lee, who observes, 'Some people are raring to go first thing in the morning, while other people won't even speak for at least half an hour after the alarm goes off. Your personal rhythm within a 24-hour period, as well as your relationship to the sun and moon, heat and cold, and the crispness or thickness of the changing seasons, can factor into which asanas you practise when. Since an important part of yoga practice is getting to know yourself and how you change from moment to moment, it makes sense to let your energy inform you about how to practise according to the season or time of day.' In other words, as with so many aspects of yoga, try out different timings – and always listen to your own body.

Don't eat beforehand I practise yoga at 8am and can't eat a thing beforehand or it makes me feel ill. You need to wait at least an hour after even the lightest snack before doing yoga, and allow about three hours to ensure a heavy meal has been digested before starting your practice. I've also found that if I'm doing an afternoon workshop, I need to eat something beforehand – so for a 2pm start, I'll eat some protein and fruit at 11am, which will sustain me without giving me indigestion. Try to tune into what works for you.

Rest if you have a heavy cold or fever A few simple, upright poses may be do-able if you've got a very mild cold, but if you've got a runny nose or a temperature, be kind to yourself and skip your class or practice. (It's kinder for those around you, too.) Go back to the mat once you're feeling better, but take a stash of tissues: any position in which your head is upside-down is likely to get your nose running again.

Stop if you feel dizzy or nauseous Also if you feel faint at any time or experience sharp pain. There's a (discernible) difference between a pain that says, 'Yes, that's really working', and one that shouts 'Uh-oh, something's wrong!' For more about ensuring that 'om' doesn't turn into 'ouch', see page 38.

Always be aware of your 'alignment' It can be hard to get this right to start with, but in yoga you should aim to align your arms, legs, torso, neck and head. If your arms are out at shoulder height, they should be evenly extended. In many poses, your head should be positioned as if it is being gently pulled up by a magnet, freeing up the neck. If you're standing, your weight should be evenly distributed through your feet – and you'll know you've got it right when you feel rooted into the earth while at the same time having a sense of weightlessness. This has only happened to me a couple of times, but on occasion I've literally felt as if I was floating above my mat in Mountain Pose (see page 60). For that moment, I knew I was in perfect alignment.

At home, it can be helpful to practise near a mirror at first so that you can see whether you're perfectly aligned. However, since I personally run a mile from yoga studios that have mirrors, and would do almost anything to avoid seeing my reflection while I'm practising, I know this isn't for everyone. So in order to get a sense of what 'alignment' feels like, try the exercise in the box right:

Just breathe Most breathing, in yoga, is done through the nose, rather than the mouth, as softly and smoothly as possible. And the 'rules' are fairly basic: pretty much every time you fold forwards towards your leg/s (such as in a forward bend) or move a limb towards you, you should exhale. Every time you lift your torso, or move a limb away from you, you should breathe in. It all feels very natural when you've done it a few times. (The only exception is if you've done a lot of Pilates, where the technique is – annoyingly – almost in reverse.) When you begin yoga, you may find yourself holding your breath – and this may crop up again when you meet any challenging pose. If this happens, then exhale slowly, and consciously try to return to steady, rhythmic breathing. In time, this will become second nature.

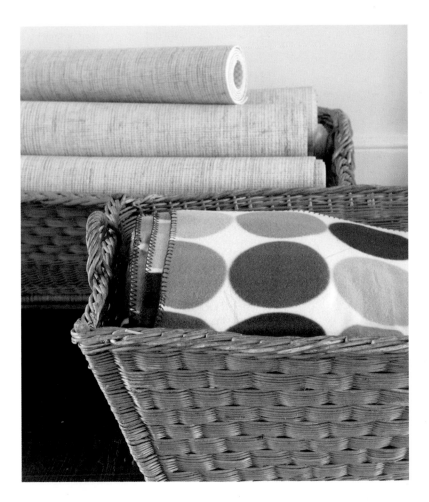

Checking your alignment

This exercise gives you a sense of what you'll feel when you get a yoga pose 'right' – then you won't need to look in a mirror to understand a pose.

1 Find a dining chair, and sit on the edge of the chair with your thighs parallel to the ground, your knees at right angles and the soles of your feet resting flat on the floor. Rest your hands on your thighs. Close your eyes and slump forward, in couch-potato mode. Stay here for a minute or two. Now straighten up and think about how that position made you feel. (Thought so.)

2 Return to your initial sitting position. Now sit up straight, feeling your spine lengthen, as if your head were being magnetised towards the ceiling. Your chin should be parallel to the floor, your neck straight. Don't strain, but sit as comfortably as you can for a minute or two. Now, how did that make you feel? Isn't the energy coursing beautifully through you now? Don't you feel tall and more powerful? This is how every yoga pose should make you feel.

Working through the poses

The postures in the book are listed first by category (Standing Pose, Inversion and so on), and then by level of difficulty within those categories. Start with Basic postures if you are new to yoga, and progress through the levels as you grow in strength, balance and confidence.

Mountain Pose (Tadasana)
STANDING: BASIC

Just how hard can it be to stand with your legs apart and your feet hip-width apart? Well, quite tricky actually. When you take up yoga, this should be the very first posture you do, and it's important to get it right from the start: it roots you firmly on your mat and a good, strong Mountain Pose sets a firm foundation for every other part of your practice. Read on to see how it can help you detect the areas where your natural posture needs attention. Mountain Pose is also the perfect antidote to all that 'living in our heads', so try to grab two minutes away from your computer screen to practise it during the day.

GOOD FOR:
- A sense of stillness
- Feeling connected with the earth
- Breathing (it improves respiration and circulation)
- Correcting postural problems

START BY: standing on your mat with your feet parallel and slightly apart. Spread your toes as far as feels comfortable and natural. Distribute your weight evenly between the front of your feet and your heels. It can be helpful to think of each foot as a tripod, with one point at each of the outer edges of the foot and a third point directly under the heel. Feel as if you have roots growing down into the earth.

1 Place your hands by your side, slightly apart from your body, fingers pointing towards the floor. Extend your fingers downwards so you feel a slight stretch in the backs of your arms.

2 Engage your feet by lifting the arches. Gently tighten your knees by pulling up your front thigh (quadriceps) muscles.

3 Let the back of your body relax slightly, and open your chest by lifting your breastbone and moving your shoulder blades gently back and down.

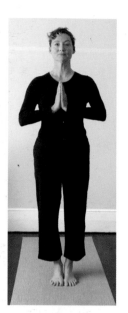

You can also finish with palms in prayer position, in front of your heart

4 Make sure your head is level and your gaze is steady. This is a pose in which you want to feel as if you have perfect posture. Stay in the pose for 4–10 breaths before relaxing.

Do...
- Imagine a string gently pulling up the top of your head, as if you were a puppet; this can help draw your head upwards.
- Relax any tension in your face and neck.
- Stay longer in the pose if you like.

Don't...
- Place your feet too far apart. Your hips are narrower than you think!
- Jut out your chin.
- Exaggerate the chest-opening; move your shoulders back gently rather than imitating a puffed-up pigeon.
- Rush.

Alternative option
For a truly centring experience, practise Mountain Pose with your feet placed firmly together and big toes touching. Then after Step 4, bring your palms together in prayer position, in front of your heart. Feel as if you are lifting your inner ankles, kneecaps and thighs. Your chin should be parallel with the floor. Release any tension from your neck and shoulders, and when you feel you're in a position of balance, gently close your eyes for a few breaths.

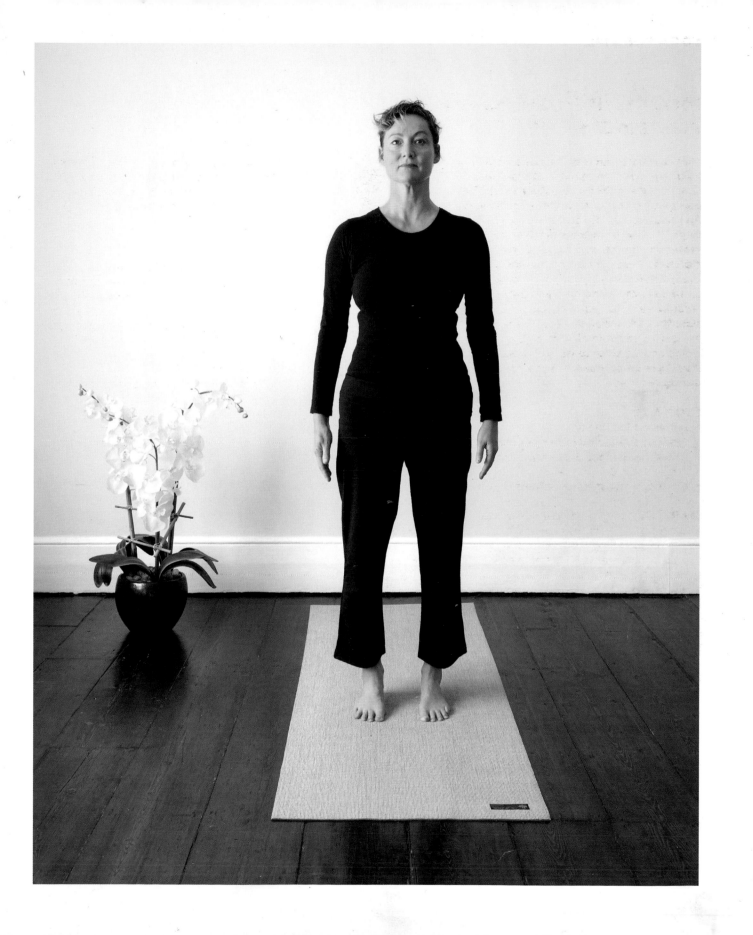

Mountain Pose with Arms Overhead (Urdhva Hastasana in Tadasana)
STANDING: BASIC

Just a slight variation on Mountain pose (which is one of the 'foundations' of yoga practice, and the starting point for so many exercises). A great one to do in the office when you've been at a screen all day, because it gives shoulders a welcome workout.

GOOD FOR:
- **Boosting energy**
- **Easing stiff and creaky shoulders**
- **Correcting postural problems**

START BY: standing on your mat in Mountain Pose (see page 60) – it's up to you whether you start with your feet slightly apart or with your toes touching.

1 Lift your arms out to the side and then up above your head, keeping them shoulder-width apart.

2 Check to make sure that your shoulders are down, away from your ears. In fact, draw your shoulder blades deep into your back, while lifting your chest.

3 Hold the pose, breathing normally, for 20–30 seconds.

4 Release your arms and let them rest gently by your sides again. Repeat the pose if you like.

Do...
- Be sure that your chin stays level and your gaze is straight ahead.

Don't...
- Hunch.

Identifying postural problems

When beginning yoga, you can use Mountain Pose to figure out which parts of your posture need special attention. It's useful to do this before trying any other poses. The aim of this exercise is simply to introduce you to your natural posture. If you find it easy to stand naturally like this, without feeling any strain or strangeness, great. If not, yoga will work on it – maybe not next week, maybe not even next month, but over time the postures can work miracles on even the creakiest, wonkiest bodies. I've seen it happen on the mat (or up against the wall), time after time.

1 Stand with your back to an unobstructed wall with your feet together (if this feels uncomfortable, separate your feet by 7–10cm). Shuffle into position so that the wall's surface is against your back. Feel your feet planted firmly on the ground. Assess the distribution of your weight: is there more weight on one side than other? Be aware that you may need to work on that.

2 Make sure that the arch of each foot is lifting and your toes are spread. Then shift your weight around a bit on your firmly rooted feet: to the front, back, left and right. Explore, becoming aware of how you actually stand.

3 Firm and straighten your legs, then lift your abdominal muscles (don't suck your tummy in). There should still be a space between the lumbar curve of your spine and the wall.

4 Lift your breastbone (without sticking out your ribs), then drop your shoulders. Open your chest and gently lift your head, as if it's being magnetised towards the ceiling without any strain. Your chin should be parallel to the floor and your gaze perfectly forward. Don't tip your head back to rest it against the wall; try to find its natural position, which is likely to be a little in front of the wall. However, do keep your shoulders resting against the wall. Hold the position for a few breaths, noticing what feels natural and where there is any tightness or strain. Then relax. Once you start practising yoga regularly, return to this pose to see how your posture is changing.

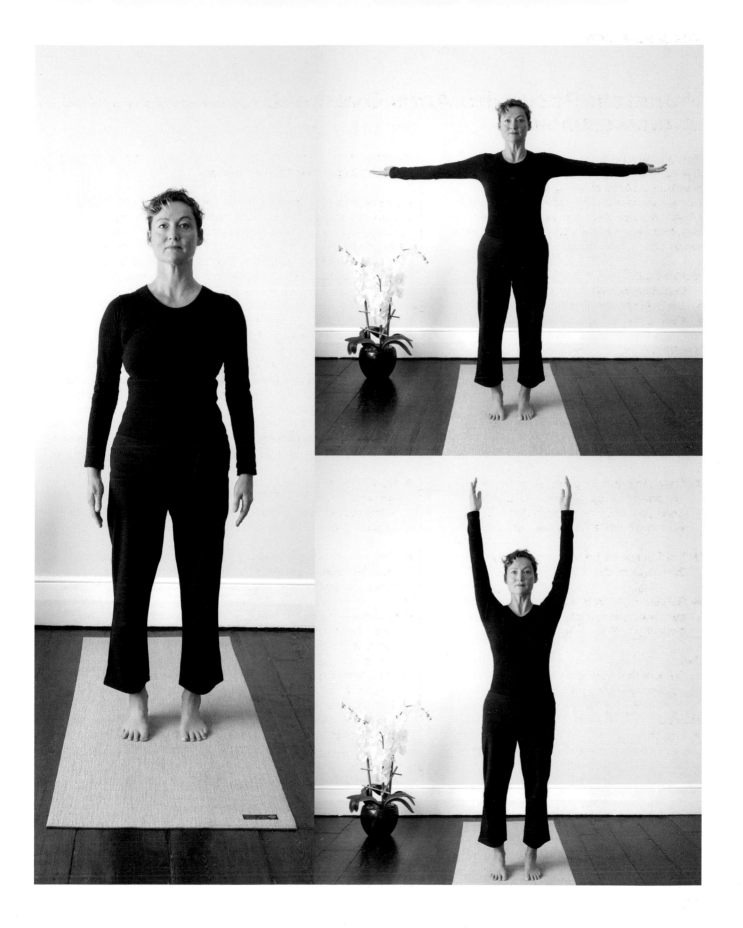

Downward-facing Dog Pose (Adho Mukha Svanasana)
STANDING: BASIC

Overall, this is considered to be one of the most beneficial of all the yoga poses; so if you don't have time for anything else each day, do find a moment for Downward Dog. This is a fantastic stretch when you've been stuck at a desk. It also brings all the benefits of a mild 'inversion' because in the pose your head is below your heart.

GOOD FOR:
- **Strengthening the hands, wrists, lower back, hamstrings, calves and Achilles tendon**
- **Back pain**
- **Decreasing anxiety**
- **Improving circulation**
- **Tension headaches (it elongates the cervical spine and relaxes the head)**

START BY: getting into 'table' position: place your knees, the top of your feet and the palms of your hands on your mat (with fingers outstretched). Keep your legs aligned and your hands shoulder-width apart; make sure your middle fingers are pointing forwards. Feel as if the base of your fingers are evenly and firmly 'rooted' into the mat.

1 Exhale and tuck your toes under; pull your lower abdominal muscles in as you push your bottom back and straighten your legs. You will now be an upside-down 'V' shape.

2 Lengthen your spine upwards and backwards.

3 With your next exhalation, lower your heels. Don't overstretch, but aim to get your heels on the ground (eventually).

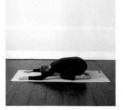

Follow with the 'counter-posture' Child Pose

4 Press firmly into your feet and hands and feel your spine lengthening.

5 Hold the pose for 5–10 long, deep breaths when you are starting out. Keep your eyes closed or look at the tip of your nose, keeping your gaze soft. When you've been doing Downward Dog for a while, you may be able to hold the position for several minutes – it's actually considered a 'resting' posture by some people.

6 To come down, slowly bend your knees and place them on the floor. Repeat, or end on the 'counter-posture' Child Pose (see page 118).

Do...
- Experiment with Downward Dog once you've got the hang of it. If your knees can take it, from 'table' position slowly lift your knees a couple of inches off the floor, initially. Push your tail backwards to lengthen your spine and then lift your belly into that 'V' position.
- Use a prop if your heels don't reach the ground. This can stop your legs from wobbling. Try slipping a flat block beneath your heels, or a thin triangular 'wedge' (see page 52). If you've always worn heels, you may never be able to get your heels flat on the ground – but a supportive block can allow you to relax into the posture.

Don't...
- Let your head hang loose; it should be relaxed but not too floppy, and in line with your spine.
- Hunch your shoulders; imagine them softening and broadening.
- Let your lower spine curve.
- Lock your elbow or knee joints.
- Stay too long in the pose if it hurts your wrists. It's better to go down, rest, then go up again.

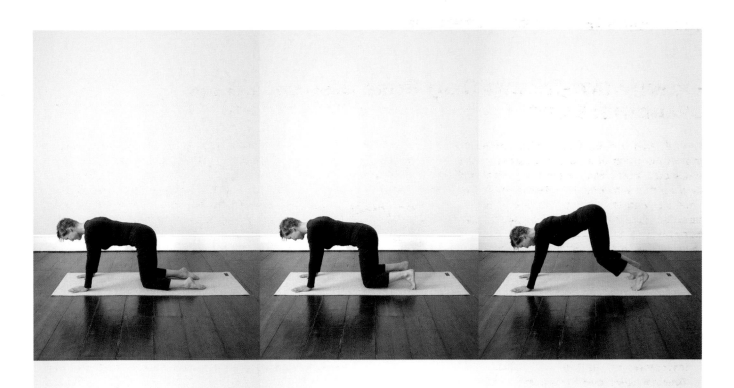

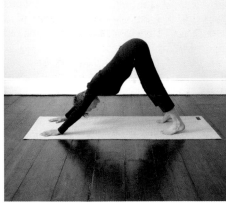

If you've always
worn heels, you
may never be able
to get your heels
flat on the ground
– but a supportive
block can allow
you to relax into
the posture

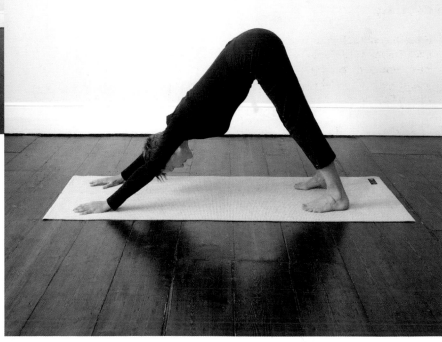

Warrior Pose I (Virabhadrasana I)
STANDING: MEDIUM

Yoga's all about non-violence – so why 'warrior'? Well, this posture's all about strength – but it's also about harmony: it requires concentration, so Warrior poses bring mind and body together in deep concentration. You'll probably wobble at first, but will become a strong warrior in no time.

GOOD FOR:
- **Sciatica**
- **Building overall strength in the arms, shoulders and back muscles**
- **Stretching and strengthening the legs**

START BY: standing in Mountain Pose (see page 60) towards the back of your mat, facing the side.

1   As you exhale, step your right foot forward by 90–120cm (depending on the length of your legs). Your front foot should face directly forward, but angle your back foot so that the toes point outwards at a 45–60 degree angle. Your heels should be in line with each other on the mat, rather than spaced more widely apart.

2   Raise your arms to shoulder level, parallel with the floor.

3   When you feel anchored in the position, breathe out and bend your front knee. If you can't see your toes, you've bent the knee too far. If you feel any twinges in your back, back off from the bend by coming up a little.

4   Gently draw in your abdominal muscles. At the same time, try to 'square' your pelvis; it's awfully easy to tilt outwards in the direction of the back leg, so consciously square your hips until (eventually) they are both facing forward.

5   Look out over your extended front arm with a soft gaze.

6   Try to hold the posture for 30 seconds (don't worry if you wobble and shake to begin with). When you are stronger and the pose starts to feel more comfortable, hold it for up to a minute.

7   To come out of Warrior I, press your back heel into the mat and straighten your right knee. Turn both feet forwards and release your arms back down to your sides, while breathing out.

8   Step back into Mountain Pose and repeat all the steps on the other side.

Do...
- Feel your shoulder blades pulling down your back.

Don't...
- Extend your knee so that it's too far forward (look at the photo opposite for the optimum angle); over-extension is bad for knees.
- Stay for long in the pose if you have blood-pressure issues. This is a strong pose that generates a lot of 'heat' in the body.
- Practise this pose if you have heart problems until you've discussed it with a qualified yoga teacher and/or with your doctor.

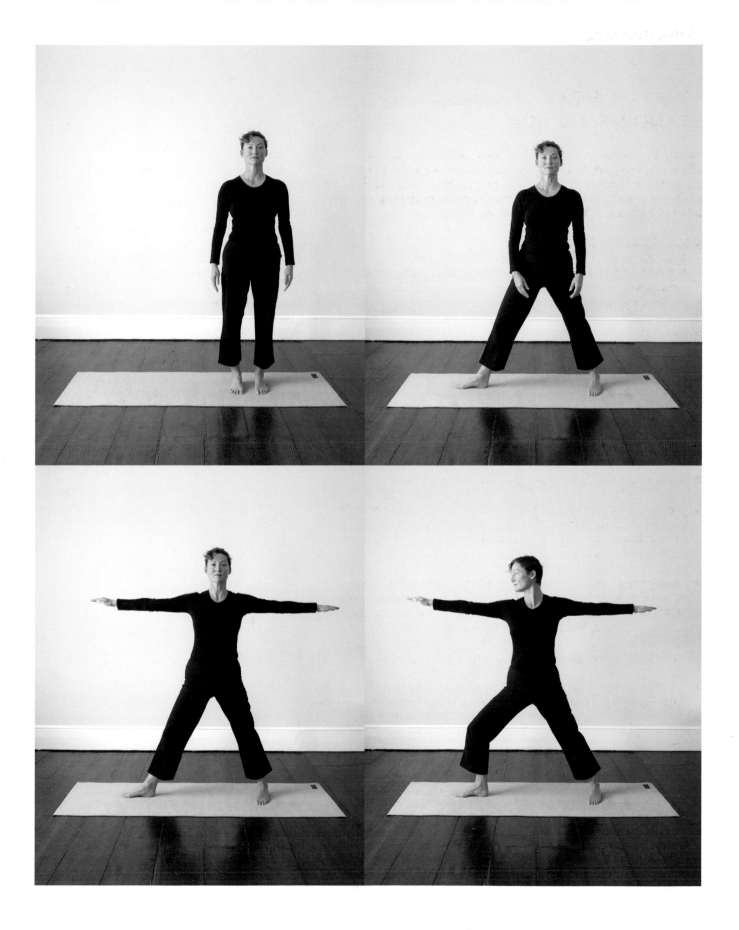

Triangle Pose (Utthita Trikonasana)
STANDING: MEDIUM

This can be a 'hated' posture in yoga, to start with (it's an unyogic concept, that, but doesn't stop people feeling it...!) Triangle is fantastic for boosting balance, but it's the wobbliness it can show up which many people find unsettling, at first. But it's amazing how swift progress can be, and props – or a wall – really help, here.

GOOD FOR:
- **Balance**
- **Stretching the muscles around the spine and trunk**
- **Invigorating the body**
- **Assisting digestion**
- **Relieving stress**

START BY: standing in Mountain Pose (see page 60), facing the long side of your mat. If needed, place a firm block near your right ankle.

1 Step your feet around 90cm apart. (If your legs are long, take your feet slightly wider apart.) Turn your right (front) foot so that it is parallel to the sides of your mat. Turn your left (back) foot in slightly.

2 Once you feel your feet are rooted into your mat, breathe in and raise your arms to shoulder-height. They should also be parallel to the long side of your mat. Rotate your shoulders slightly towards each other, firming your arms and extending them as far as you can through the tips of your fingers. Enjoy that stretch!

3 Keeping your legs firm and strong, extend the right arm forward. Hinge at the right hip, without twisting your torso. Then bring your hand to rest either on a block or (if you're more flexible) on your ankle, the top of your foot or the floor. Rest your hand lightly, rather than dropping your full weight down onto your wrist; your legs and waist should be doing all the support work.

4 Raise your left arm directly above your shoulder towards the ceiling. It should point strongly upwards, towards the sky – if your body were a clock, your upper arm would be at precisely 12 o'clock.

5 Gaze straight ahead (softly), to start with. When, with practice, you start to feel well balanced in this posture, you can turn your head to look at your skywards hand.

6 To come out of the pose, bend your front knee as you bring your torso up, hinging from your front hip. Raise your arms to shoulder-height before dropping them back down to your sides.

7 Move the block, if used, near your left ankle and repeat all the steps on that side.

Do...
- Focus on alignment. Try this pose, initially, against a wall to learn how it feels to be perfectly 'straight', rather than tipping forwards or leaning back. In fact, if you feel nervous about your balance in this pose, always practise against a wall until you feel more secure.
- Imagine your feet have four corners, and distribute your weight evenly over all four corners of each foot to help you balance.
- Try visualising a huge bird (like an albatross) floating on a current of air, with its wings outstretched; this can help you maintain a strong posture.
- Keep the front of your pelvis open – 'smiling', as some teachers put it.
- Remember to breathe deeply and rhythmically.
- Turn to look at your top hand once you feel well balanced in the posture.

Don't...
- Let the outer edge of your feet collapse outwards.
- Cheat by dropping your weight into the hand resting on your leg, the block or the ground. Let it rest lightly, so that you're strengthening your core.
- Position your lower arm on your knee, which will strain it. Thigh, yes; calf/ankle, yes, but no pressure on the knee ever.
- Drop your eyes floorwards; they should gaze either ahead or up at your hand.

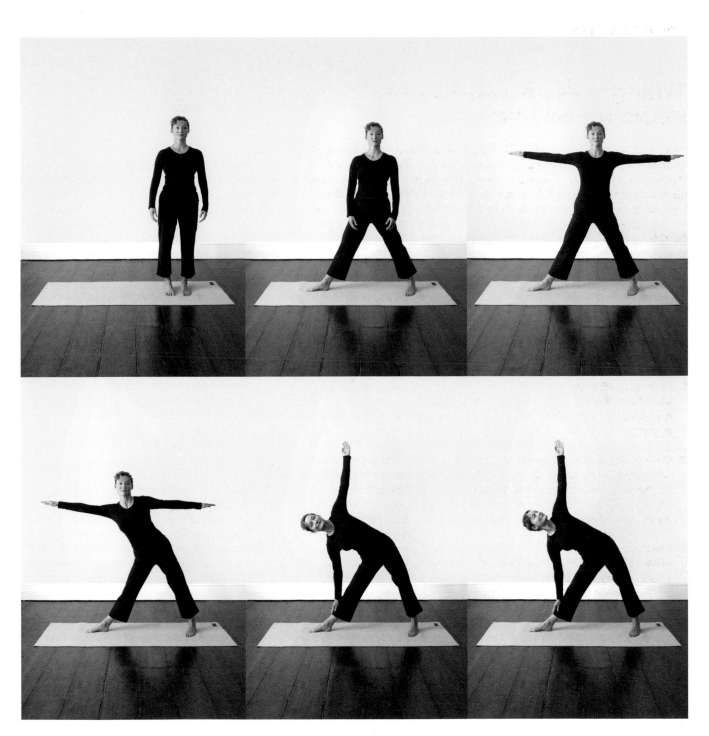

Triangle is fantastic for boosting balance,
but it's the wobbliness it can reveal which
many people find unsettling, at first

Tree Pose (Vrkasana)
BALANCING: BASIC

This is a terrific posture for helping to prevent you from falling over like a ninepin later in life. It is also said in yoga circles that if you practise Tree Pose regularly, your mind will become as strong as an oak tree. Be kind to yourself when practising this pose; to start with everyone wobbles like crazy, but Tree Pose is amazingly strengthening and it really does get easier, with time, to stay in the pose. It's also natural for this pose to feel easier on one side than the other.

GOOD FOR:
• **Strengthening the legs**
• **Improving concentration and balance**
• **Improved breathing**

START BY: placing your mat beside a wall, for support, or next to the back of a chair, with the seat facing away from you. You don't have to use either, but when you start learning this pose, it's reassuring to know they're there.

1 Stand in Mountain Pose (see page 60), with your feet hip-width apart and facing forwards. Make sure your weight is evenly distributed between your feet.

2 Transfer your weight to your right foot and raise your left foot.

3 Once you can balance steadily, raise your left knee towards your chest and gently clasp the outside with both hands, one on top of the other. Engage your abdominal muscles and feel your lower back lengthen. Make sure you are breathing deeply and smoothly to aid your balance.

4 There are variations at this point. If you're a beginner, place the sole of your right foot just above the ankle on the inside of your right leg. If you are a little more advanced, place the sole of your foot on your calf. Hold onto the chair or wall for support, if you need it. Just practise to this point (on both legs) until you have found your balance in this position and no longer need a wall or chair for support.

5 Find a drishti (or focus-point) – something that doesn't move. This will help you maintain balance. Breathe evenly through your nose as you hold the pose for a few breaths.

6 Lower your left leg to the ground; shake it if necessary to release any tension. Return to Mountain Pose, then repeat all the steps on the other leg.

Advanced option
When you are more advanced in your practice, position the sole of your left foot on your right inner thigh after step 4. It can be helpful to take hold of your right ankle and lift it into place. Your right knee should turn out by 90 degrees, and your hips be wide and 'open'. The best way to stop your foot from slipping from this raised position – and to maintain balance – is to be sure that you're pressing firmly into the opposite thigh through the sole of your raised foot. Once the raised leg and your balance feel secure, bring your palms into prayer position in front of your chest. In time, try raising your hands above your head, either in prayer position or with your arms shoulder-width apart, fingers pointing straight at the ceiling.

Do...
• Try rolling up the leg of your yoga pants or leggings, if you find that the fabric makes your foot slip.
• Lick the palm of your hand and smooth it against the sole of whichever foot you're raising; the moisture helps the foot to stay in place. (This tip is slightly 'eeewww', but it works.)
• Ditch one mat, if you tend to do yoga with two mats positioned one on top of the other. That extra springiness can make you wobble in this pose.

Don't...
• Choose another student as your 'focus point' when you're locating a place at which to gaze; it's guaranteed that when he or she wobbles, so will you.
• Feel shy about using the wall or a chair for balance.
• Place the sole of your foot against the opposite knee. This puts too much pressure on the joint. Position your sole just above the ankle, on your calf or thigh only.

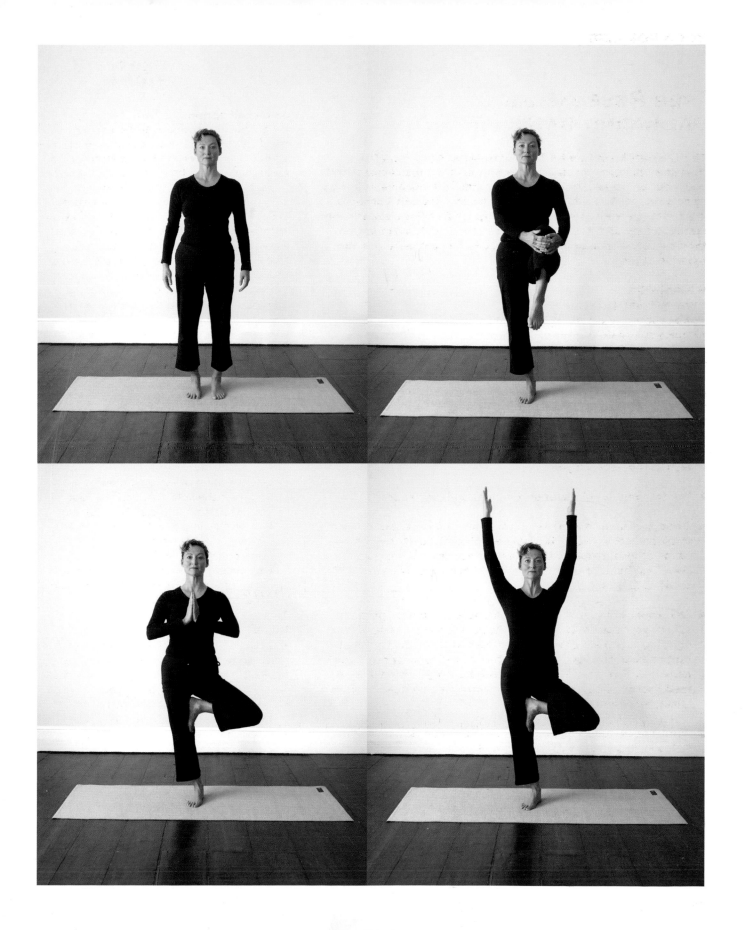

Eagle Pose (Garudasana)
BALANCING: MEDIUM DIFFICULTY

You almost 'macramé' yourself into this balancing posture, wrapping your limbs around each other. But it's fantastic for balance and focus, and is a great shoulder stretch, again, for computer-users.

GOOD FOR:
- **Improving shoulder flexibility**
- **Stretching the upper back and shoulders**
- **Balance**
- **Concentration**
- **Strengthening the knees (see warning, right, if you have knee trouble)**

START BY: standing tall on your mat in Mountain Pose (see page 60), with your feet and legs pressed together. You should feel as if the crown of your head is being lifted by a thread.

1 Maintaining your tall stance, take your weight onto your left foot. Bend your knee slightly and cross your right thigh over the standing thigh, hooking your foot behind your calf or the ankle if you can. Direct your toes towards the floor, and be sure you have your balance before moving on.

2 Stretch your arms forwards so that your left arm is above the right, then bend your elbows.

3 Tuck your left elbow into the crook of your right elbow, and raise your forearms to shoulder-height, level with the floor. The backs of your palms may be facing each other, or – if you're more flexible – you may curl your right hand around your left wrist and tuck it there, in a deeper 'spiral'. Whichever version you go for, try to keep your palms as straight as possible, fingers pointing towards the ceiling.

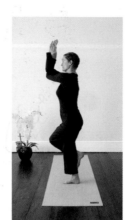

This is fantastic for balance and focus, and is a great shoulder stretch for computer-users

4 Hold the pose for 15–30 seconds or so, then unfurl gracefully and in a controlled way. It's easy to 'collapse' out of this pose, so try to keep it smooth.

5 Return to Mountain Pose, then repeat the steps on the other side, reversing everything so that the opposite leg and arm are 'on top'.

Do...
- Keep your arms at shoulder height when they are crossed, rather than allowing them to droop.
- Remember that the arm on top is the opposite one to the leg on top. So if your left leg is over your right leg, your right arm should be over your left arm. And vice versa.

Don't...
- Do this if you have any kind of knee injury or ongoing knee pain.

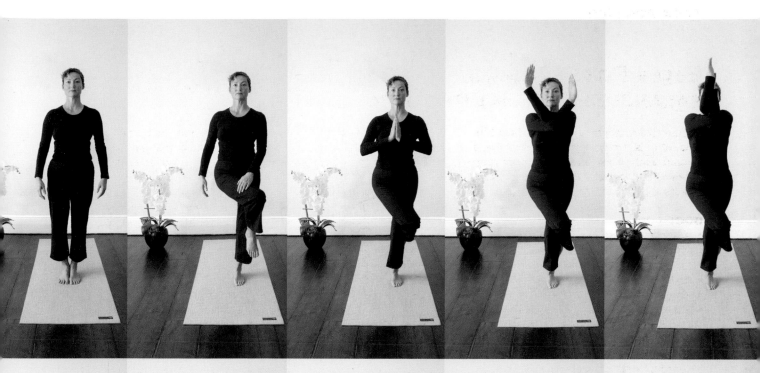

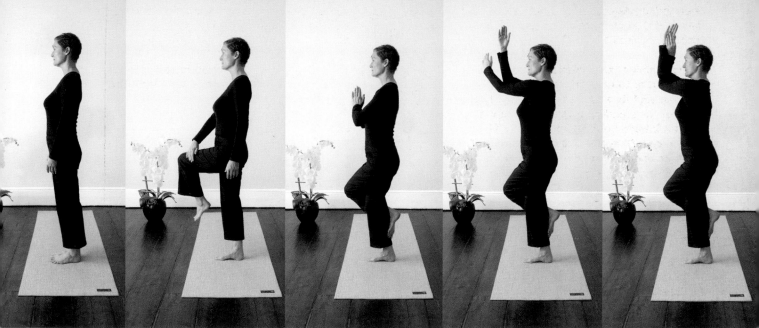

One-legged Downward-facing Dog Pose

(Eka Pada Adho Mukha Svanasana)
STANDING/BALANCING: MEDIUM DIFFICULTY

This is what I'd call a 'Stage 2' posture, and makes a wonderful addition to your practice when you've gained in confidence. According to yoga experts, this is an Americanisation: a westernised 'tweak' to Downward Dog, adding the challenge of balancing on one leg while extending the opposite.

GOOD FOR:
- **Strengthening the arms and legs**
- **Developing balance**
- **Allowing the brain to rest**

START BY: getting into Downward-facing Dog Pose (see page 64) with both palms and both feet on your mat. Your middle fingers should be facing forwards.

1 Step your left leg slightly towards your right leg, creating a 'tripod' support for the next step.

2 Press down evenly with your hands and lift your right leg off the floor, using the power of the quadriceps muscles in your thighs. Don't just 'kick' your leg into this pose, or you'll twist at the hips. Take your leg as high as you can without tilting or twisting your pelvis.

3 Feel that your weight is balanced evenly through your two hands and your standing leg. You should also feel your pelvis and sitting bones stretching away from your ribcage.

Focus on keeping your hips and pelvis 'square'. It's easy to tilt the hip out of alignment in this pose

4 Keep your foot flexed and active, and have a sense that the ball of the foot is stretching towards the wall behind you.

5 You can progress easily from this into Pigeon Pose (see page 96). Alternatively, return your foot to the ground in Downward Dog, and then drop down into Child Pose (see page 118) to give yourself a rest.

6 After resting in Child Pose for a minute or so, lift back up into Downward Dog and repeat the steps to lift your other leg.

Do...
- Focus on keeping your hips and pelvis 'square'. It's really easy to tilt the hip out of alignment in this pose.
- Feel that your leg is an extension of your spine – this is the key to maintaining good balance in the pose.
- Keep your head in line with your spine; don't tilt it to look up.

Don't...
- Point your toes; the raised foot should be flexed throughout.

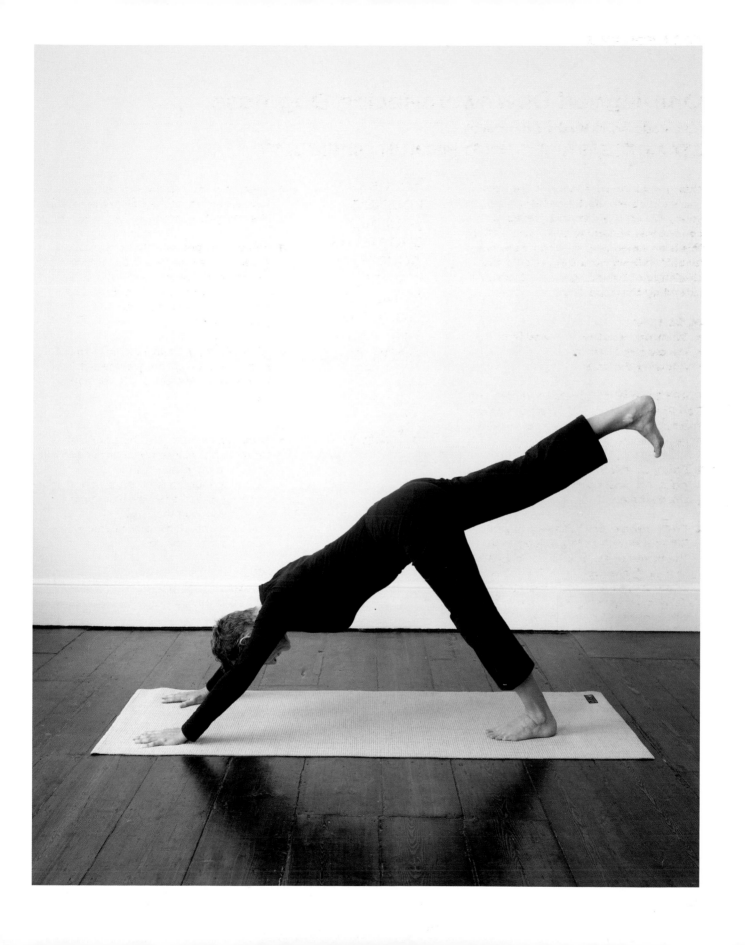

Cat Pose (Marjari Asana)
CORE STRENGTHENING: BASIC

It really does help to imagine a cat while you're doing this pose! It's a terrific stretch for the spine – great for any time you're feeling 'crunched up' from sitting – and it's also a brilliant warm-up exercise for any yoga practice, at home.

GOOD FOR:
- **Massaging the abdominal organs**
- **Learning to co-ordinate movement and breath – the heart of a yoga practice**
- **Loosening the spine**
- **Managing stress**

START BY: getting into 'table' position on your mat: place your palms beneath your shoulders, with your middle fingers pointing straight ahead. Position your knees directly under your hips, with your toes pointing towards the back of the mat. Your back should be horizontal and flat, your pelvis in a neutral position, and your gaze directed at the floor. Once you feel comfortable here, you're ready to move on.

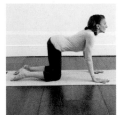

This is a terrific spine stretch– great for when you feel 'crunched up' from sitting

1 Breathe deeply. Feel as if you're creating a line of energy from your hands to your shoulders by pressing through the palms of your hands.

2 As you inhale, keep your pelvis in the same place but round your back upwards so that the middle lifts towards the ceiling. You'll now be gazing at the floor between your knees.

3 Then you exhale, gently pull your abdominal muscles backwards towards your spine, tucking your tailbone (coccyx) down and under, and gently contracting your buttocks. Be sure to keep your shoulders lifted, and look straight ahead. Find a spot a few feet ahead for your eyes to rest on. Don't tilt your head back too far.

4 As you exhale, release your shoulders to return to the flat table position. Repeat the movement a few times, co-ordinating it with your breath. Then rest in Child Pose (see page 118) if you wish.

Do...
- Place a folded blanket under your knees and feet if the floor feels too hard or the mat is scratchy on the tops of your feet.

Don't...
- Sag into your shoulders.
- Exaggerate the pose by over-arching your neck when you're exhaling and curving upwards.

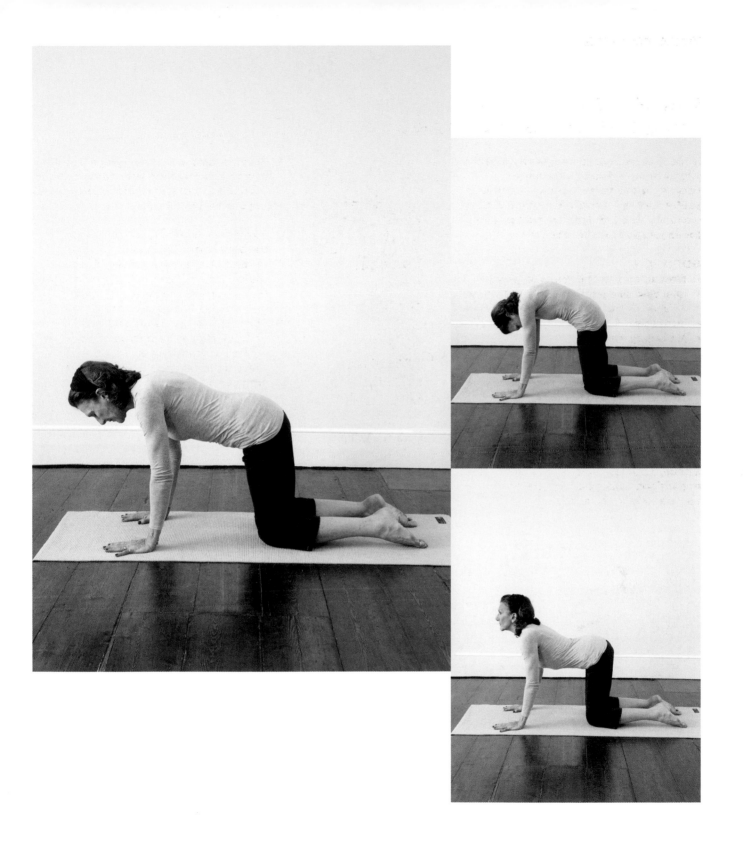

Happy Baby Pose (Ananda Balasana)
CORE STRENGTHENING: BASIC/MEDIUM DIFFICULTY

Get yourself into this pose when you've been sitting for a long time in a chair. (Although possibly not in a crowded office, and only wearing stretchy clothing...) It definitely gets rid of any creakiness. Happy Baby recreates the carefree pose of a baby lying on its back with legs akimbo; it can actually feel quite vulnerable to do this, at first, but it's such a great hip exercise – and so soothing for the mind – that you'll soon get over it.

GOOD FOR:
• **Opening the hips**
• **Releasing the lower back**
• **Calming the brain**
• **Easing fatigue and stress**

START BY: lying on your back on your mat.

1 As you exhale, bend your knees into your chest.

2 Inhale, then lift your legs and open your knees, bringing them towards your armpits.

3 Stack your lower legs so that your ankles are directly above your knees; the soles of your feet should be parallel with the ceiling.

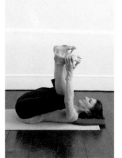

Happy Baby recreates the carefree pose of a baby lying on its back with legs akimbo

4 Flex your feet and grab hold of the outer edges of each foot. You may have to lift your head off the mat to reach your feet, but then return it to a lying position, sinking your upper back into the mat. Putting pressure on your feet with your hands, draw your knees towards the floor.

5 Hold steadily for 30 seconds, building up to a minute as you become more experienced.

Do...
• Use a folded blanket under your head if you have any neck issues. The key to this pose is not to strain your neck.
• Be careful if you have a history of knee injuries. Only do as much as is comfortable. If you feel any kind of strain, give this pose a miss.

Don't...
• Strain to grab hold of your feet. If your feet are too much of a stretch away, loop a belt around the arch of each foot and hold the ends taut.

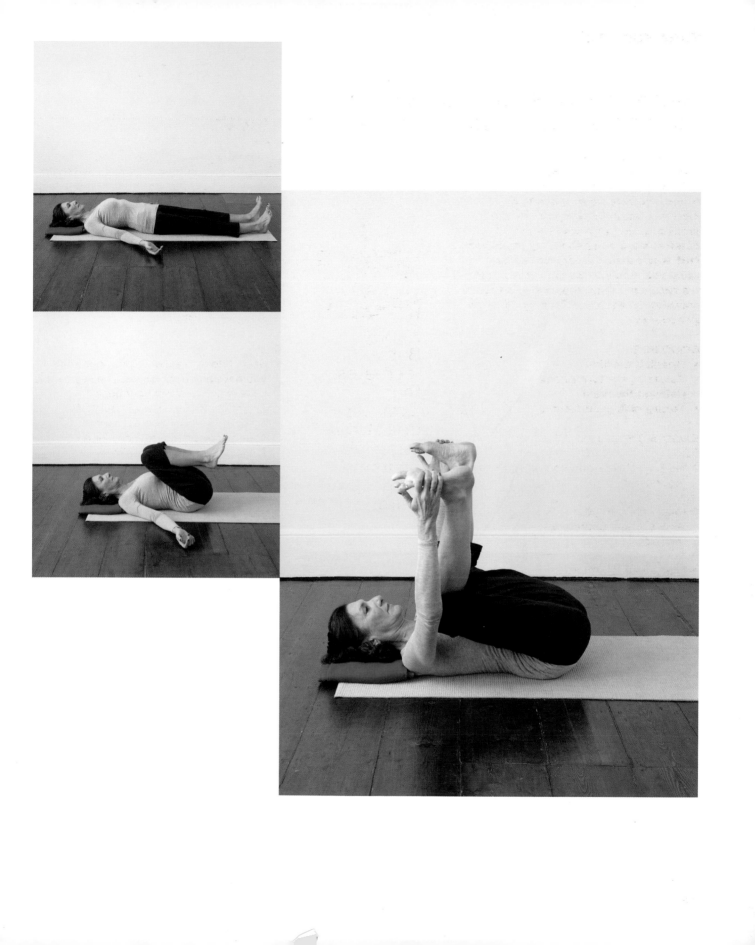

Standing Forward Bend (Uttanasana)
FORWARD BENDING: BASIC

This is a fabulous stretch in itself, but forward bends as a whole are just brilliant for spine flexibility, even if you feel stiff as a ramrod when you first try the pose. Be aware that men usually have much, much tighter hamstrings than women, and can find this pose very challenging indeed.

GOOD FOR:
- **The whole digestive system, helping to remove toxins from the body**
- **Stimulating the spine and invigorating the nervous system**
- **Boosting blood flow to the brain, aiding concentration**

START BY: standing on your mat in Mountain Pose (see page 60), with your feet slightly apart. Place a block in front of you if your hands don't easily reach the floor, to rest them on.

1 On an in-breath, lift your arms over your head, keeping your palms apart and facing each other. Be sure to keep your shoulders relaxed.

2 On an out-breath, gently fold forwards – not from the waist, but from your hip sockets. Place your hands on the floor or block in front of you, or if you are more flexible, softly clasp your legs.

3 Once you're at full reach – and only then – relax the top half of your body towards the floor slightly. Don't hunch, or your breathing will feel more constricted. With each breath, lift and lengthen your torso slightly, which allows you to drop a little further into the bend.

4 Let your head hang down. Feel as if it's dropping from the root of your neck, which is actually between your shoulder blades.

5 Start by staying in the forward bend for a few seconds, and over time, build up to a minute. Be aware that if you're not used to putting your head below your knees, you may experience a head-rush.

6 When you want to come out of the posture, bend your knees slightly, gently pull in your abdominal muscles and hinge upwards slowly from the hips.

Easier variation
If your hamstrings are really tight and you can't get your hands on the floor, either take them to a block or keep your knees slightly bent and grab hold of your opposite elbows with your hands and just 'hang'. For more support, let your folded arms rest on your thighs.

Advanced variation
If your hands easily reach the floor, lift your toes and the balls of your feet and slide your hands underneath, then lower your feet on top. Alternatively, try another traditional hand position by hooking the forefinger and thumb of each hand around the corresponding big toe.

Do...
- Experiment with placing a block on its end or on its side – whichever helps most – if you can't reach the floor with your hands.
- Keep your jaw and tongue relaxed.
- Ensure that your weight is evenly distributed between both feet, and between the front and back, left and right sides of each foot.

Don't...
- Strain to reach the floor, if the extension in the backs of your legs doesn't come easily, nor strain to bring your head closer to your knees. Over time, your hamstrings will lengthen beautifully and naturally and you'll get closer than you are now. But in the meantime, repeat the 'it's-not-a-competition' mantra.
- Allow your back to round, or slump into the posture.

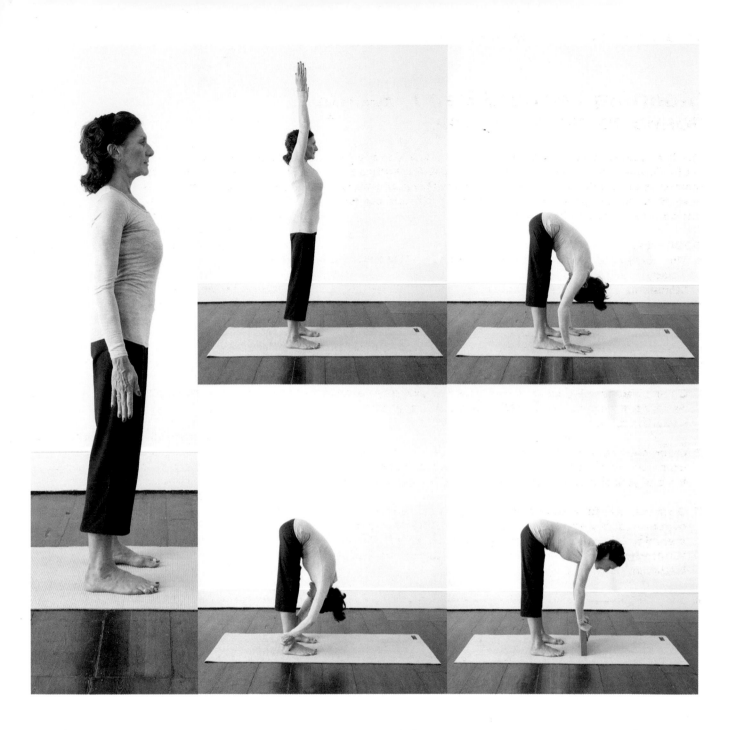

Seated Forward Bend (Paschimottanasana)
FORWARD BENDING: BASIC

The ancient texts say that this pose is good for reducing obesity! Actually, Seated Forward Bend is a bit of an all-round wonder-pose, working on many of the internal organs and body systems and even relieving mild depression.

GOOD FOR:
- **Soothing and calming the brain**
- **Stimulating the organs (liver, kidneys, female reproductive organs)**
- **Improving digestion**
- **Relieving high blood pressure and insomnia**

START BY: sitting on your mat with a folded blanket placed beneath your 'sitting bones', for support.

1 Straighten your legs in front of you. Actively press down through your heels and thighs. Place your hands or fingertips on the floor beside your hips and lift your crown as if it were being pulled up by a piece of string. (This will also lift your sternum.) This position is known as Staff Pose (see page 112).

2 Breathe in, and, keeping the front of your body nice and long, lift your arms above your head and lean forward from the hips (not your waist). Feel your tailbone lengthening.

3 Where you go from here depends on the flexibility of the hamstring muscles at the back of your thighs. If they're tight (and men in particular are prone to this), simply rest your hands on the calves, on the outside of your legs. If you are more flexible, grasp the sides of your feet, with elbows fully extended.

4 Every time you breathe out, try to lift and lengthen your torso a little more. Do not pull yourself into position, just lengthen into it from the hips. Very flexible people will be able to rest the belly, the ribs and finally the head on the legs, but most of us never, ever get to that stage.

Seated Forward Bend is an all-round wonder-pose, working on many of the internal organs and body systems and even relieving mild depression

5 Breathing deeply and evenly through your nose, stay in the position for 30 seconds at first, building up to a couple of minutes as you feel more comfortable in the pose.

6 To come out of the pose, lift your upper body by pulling your tailbone down, at the back, while engaging your abdominals. If your tummy muscles are pretty lax, there is no shame in pushing yourself up with your arms, while your abs are getting stronger.

Do...
- Loop a belt around the balls of your feet, hold the ends in your hands and pull to help lengthen your upper body forwards, if you can't get very far. As you get more comfortable in the pose, gradually walk your hands down the strap to nudge yourself deeper into the posture.
- Keep your head raised so that the crown of your head is in line with your spine.
- Place a rolled-up blanket under your knees if you are stiff or have knee problems.

Don't...
- Round your back and let your head go unless your whole upper body is resting on your thighs.
- Try this pose if you are asthmatic. (It can feel sometimes as if your breath is being restricted.)
- Go into a seated forward bend if you have a back injury, unless you are supervised by a really experienced teacher who knows about your problem.

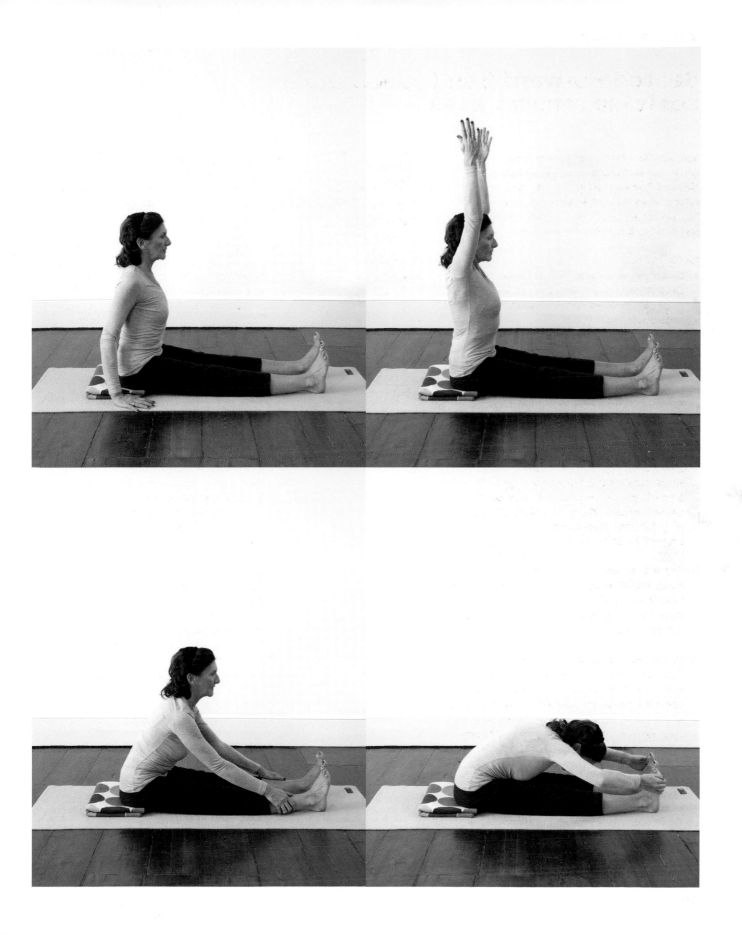

Wide-legged Forward Bend (Prasarita Padottanasana)
FORWARD BENDING: BASIC

This is a posture which (in a class) can make anyone with tight hamstrings feel truly like a beginner, perhaps only able to reach an upturned block (while other classmates can even get their elbows on the ground...) Progress is rapid, though, and this is brilliantly grounding and brain-soothing: as good for your grey matter as those taut hamstrings.

GOOD FOR:
- **Strengthening and stretching the inner thighs and backs of the legs, plus the spine**
- **Relieving headaches**
- **Countering tiredness**
- **Easing mild backache**

START BY: standing in Mountain Pose (see page 60), turned sideways on your mat so that you are facing the long side rather than the narrow front of the mat. Move your feet towards the back of the mat.

1 Step your legs apart and your feet parallel with one another. Ultimately, your feet should be the same distance apart as your wrists would be if you straightened your arms sideways. But to begin with, be far less ambitious!

2 Rest your hands on your hips. Draw up the inner arches of your feet and press the outer edges down into the mat. (It's amazing, after a while, how you gain control of individual muscles in your feet!)

3 Engage your thigh muscles, breathe in and lift your chest.

4 Hinge forward from your hip joints, leaning your torso forwards. When your upper body is parallel to the floor, place your fingertips on the floor, directly below your shoulders, and extend your elbows (but don't lock them). Alternatively, if you are flexible enough, place your palms flat on the floor, fingers facing forwards. Keep your

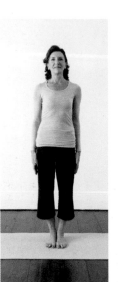

Start by: standing in Mountain Pose, turned sideways on your mat

head in line with the rest of your spine and allow your eyes to gaze softly at the floor. Hold the pose for a few breaths, breathing normally.

5 To come out of the pose, breathe in, place your hands on your hips, bend your knees slightly and swing your upper body upwards, pulling your tailbone towards the floor. Then step your feet together into Mountain Pose.

6 Repeat, if you choose, building up the amount of time you spend in this pose.

Advanced variation
If and when you are flexible enough, try moving to the next stage after step 4. Walk your fingertips sideways and back between your feet, or perhaps even rest them on top of your feet, if you're very bendy. Breathe deeply, then bend your elbows and lower your upper body and head into a full forward bend. If possible, rest the crown of your head on the floor. Only do this when you really feel truly ready!

Do...
- Rest your hands on a block in front of you, placed either flat on the floor or on its end, if your hands don't easily reach the floor. Or try two blocks, one under each hand. Experiment to see what gives you optimum support.
- Be aware that this pose can make you feel dizzy, so if you have high or low blood pressure, take it really easy and be especially careful coming up.

Don't...
- Sink down so that all your weight is on your hands: this places pressure on your wrists. In a perfect world, you should have your tummy muscles engaged so that if you took your hands off the floor, you could maintain the same position.
- Come up with straight or locked knees, which puts too much pressure on them.

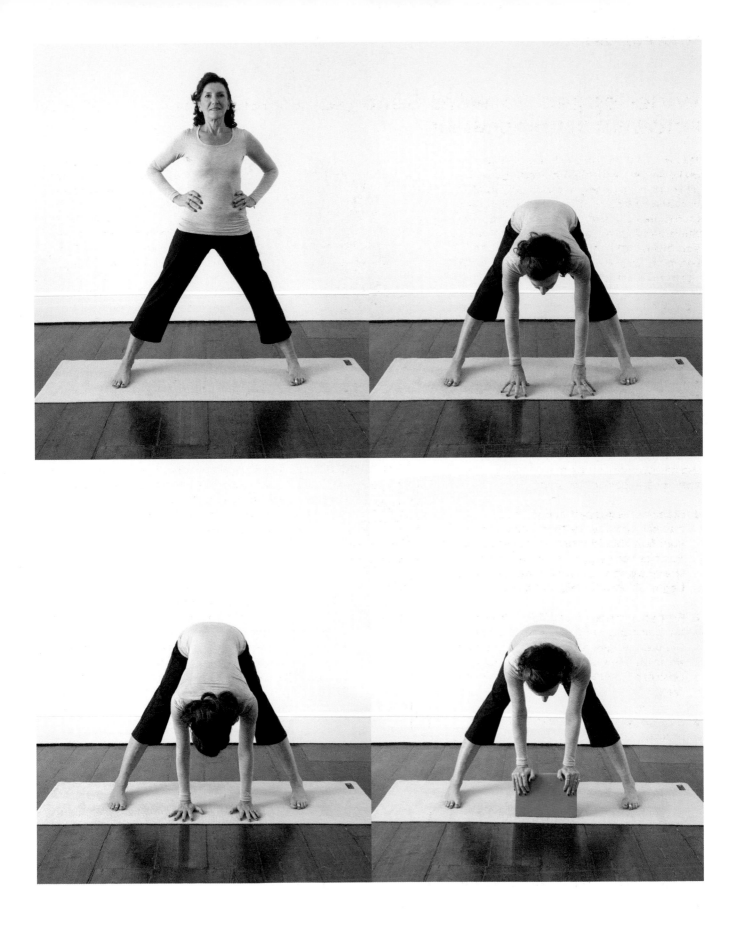

Big Toe Pose (Padangusthasana)
FORWARD BENDING: INTERMEDIATE

Another fantastic posture for stretching out tight hamstrings, but this offers so much more than just a thigh workout: it is great for finding your 'roots', making you feel more grounded both on and off the mat. Unless you're super-flexible, you could secretly rename this: 'Hands-on-a-strap' pose, because it will feel as if you'll never actually hook those fingers under your toes – but with practice, it's amazing how you'll edge gradually towards the mat.

GOOD FOR:
- **Easing menopausal symptoms**
- **Countering osteoporosis**
- **Calming the brain and relieving stress and anxiety**
- **Improving digestion**
- **Relieving headaches**

START BY: standing on your mat in Mountain Pose (see page 60), with your feet parallel and about 15cm apart. Lift your kneecaps by contracting the muscles at the front of your thighs.

1 Exhale and hinge forward from your hip joints, keeping your head and torso in line.

2 Slide your first and middle fingers under your big toes, and curl them around to meet your thumbs. Take a firm grip. Use a strap if you can't easily hook your fingers around your big toes (see right).

3 Breathe in, and lift your chest and head as if you were going to stand up again. Straighten your elbows.

Use a belt if you can't touch your toes. It's more important to keep your legs straight than to reach your toes

4 Maintain this position, but on your next exhalation, feel as if you're 'lifting' your sitting bones. Lift your belly, at the same time, towards the back of your pelvis. As you lift your sitting bones you'll feel a stretch in your hamstrings and calves.

5 Repeat the following very subtle movements over the next few in- and out-breaths: as you inhale, lift your chest, being careful not to tip your head backwards; on the exhalation, lift your sitting bones.

6 Exhale one more time, bend your elbows and gently lower your torso into a full forward bend. Stay here for up to a minute (you can build up to this).

7 Release your toes, bring your hands to your hips and swing your torso upright. Bend your knees a little as you come up.

Do...
- Place your hands on your hips initially, as you hinge forwards, if you feel you need a little extra support.
- Keep your knees straight when you're in the pose.
- Use a belt if you can't touch your toes (it's more important to keep your legs straight than to reach your toes). Hook the belt around the balls of your feet before you start, then grab the belt instead of your toes. Keep the straps taut.

Don't...
- 'Curl' or hunch as you lean forward; your torso and head should be a single unit. The focus should be on keeping the front of your torso long.

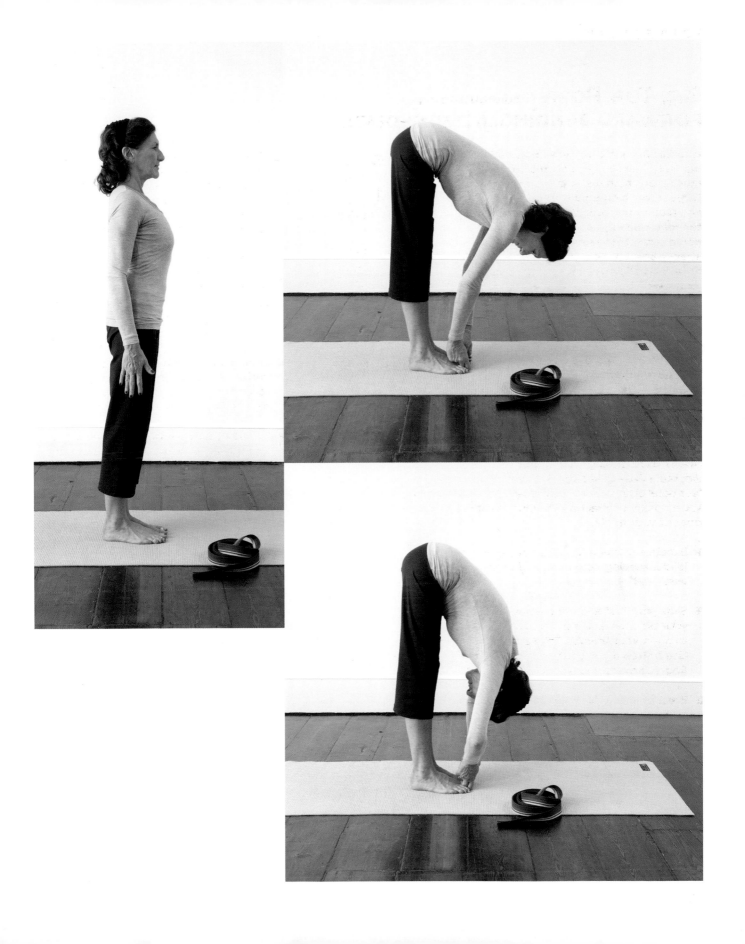

Cobbler Pose (Baddha Konasana)
FORWARD BENDING: MEDIUM DIFFICULTY

Some teachers refer to this posture as
'Bound Angle Pose'.

GOOD FOR:
- **Opening the hips and groin**
- **Stimulating the abdominal organs**
- **Relieving menopausal symptoms**

START BY: sitting on your mat with your
legs straight out in front of you – this is
known as Staff Pose (see page 112).

1 Bend your knees, bringing the soles
of your feet together and letting your
knees fall out to either side.

2 Straighten your back so that you are
sitting tall.

3 Firmly press the outer edges of your feet
together.

4 Hook your thumbs and forefingers
around your big toe, or if that's too
difficult, grasp your ankles or calves.

5 As you get more advanced in this pose,
lean forwards with your torso, keeping
your back straight and your head in line
with your spine, for a fantastic groin
stretch.

6 Hold the pose for one minute, building
up to five minutes, as your practice
progresses.

Do...
- Loop a belt around your feet and hold
onto the ends, keeping the strap taut,
if you are not comfortable holding your
feet or legs.

Don't...
- Let your back curve or hunch when you
are leaning forwards.

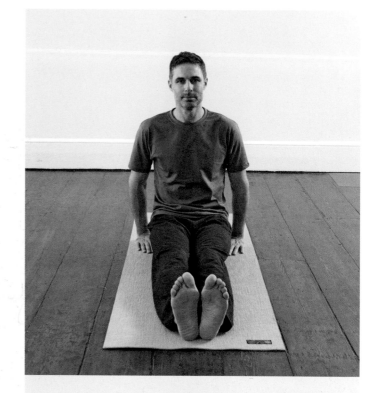

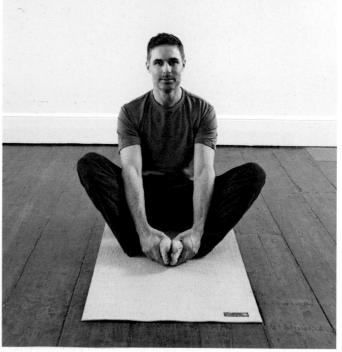

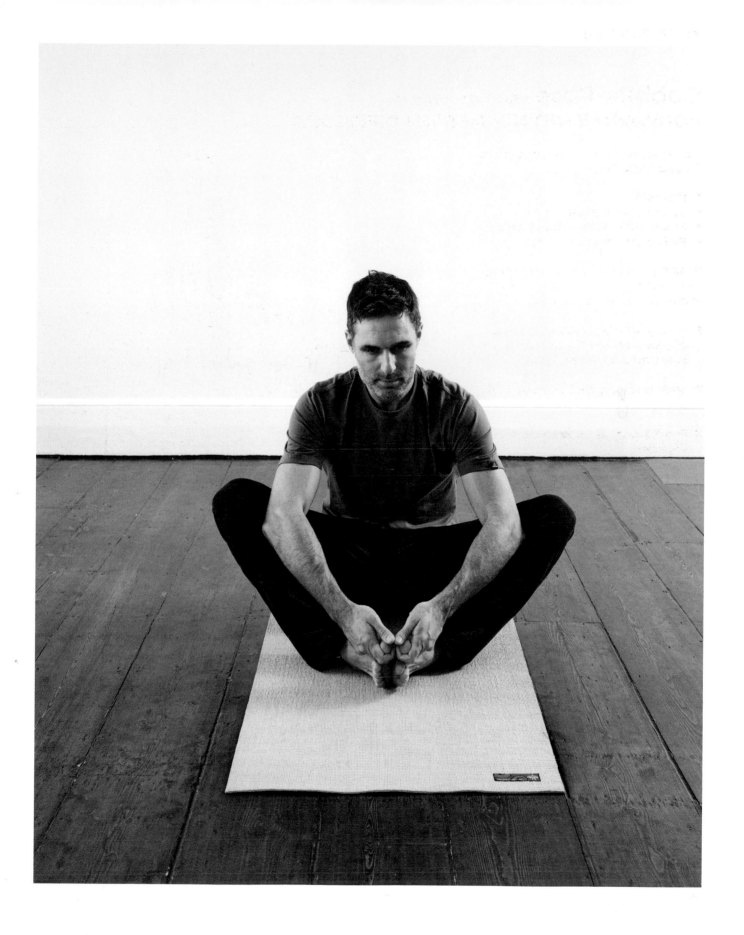

Sphinx Pose (Salamba Bhujangasana)
BACKBENDING: BASIC

This is a gentle introduction to backbends, including Cobra. Backbends can't be rushed: you need to get the body used to them gently, because it's such an unfamiliar position in our forward-hunched lives (think: computers, iPads, books). You're literally recreating the pose of the Egyptian sphinx statues, here.

GOOD FOR:
• **Relieving stress**
• **Strengthening the spine**
• **Stimulating the internal organs (reproductive, digestive)**
• **Preparing for Cobra Pose (see page 94)**

START BY: lying on your tummy, with your legs side-by-side, arms bent at shoulder-height and fingers pointing to the front of your mat.

1 Reach your toes back behind you. Your buttocks should be firm, but not over-tightened. Actively relax your eyes, tongue and mind.

2 Slide your hands and forearms forwards. Press down through your elbows and forearms while gently using your abdominal muscles to lift your torso and head up from the floor, in a 'baby' backbend.

3 Look at the wall straight ahead of you with a soft gaze. Keep your abdominal muscles engaged but not clenched.

4 Stay in the pose for three or four breaths, building up to ten breaths over time as you become more experienced.

5 Exhale, then gradually release your abdominal muscles and lower your head and torso to the floor in one smooth movement. Turn your head to one side. Rest for a little while, sinking into the mat.

6 Repeat the steps; when you return to the mat the second time, turn your head to the opposite side to rest. Repeat a few times to build up strength, turning your head in alternate directions to rest each time.

Do...
• Only lift your upper body a few centimetres off the floor, if that's all that's comfortable. Stop and lower yourself if there is any hint of pinching in your lower spine.
• Place a thin folded blanket under your pubic bone, if you find this area presses uncomfortably into the mat.

Don't...
• Tip your head backwards.
• Try this pose (or any backbends) if you have a back injury. Consult your doctor or physiotherapist for further advice.

A word on boobs

Yoga was invented by men, no question. They did not have to tussle with breasts in yoga postures. (OK, so men have other anatomical challenges, but they're on a smaller scale. Mostly.) Although a good sports bra can help keep your breasts in place, be aware that you may have to make small adjustments to postures if you are generously endowed in the bust department.

You may also have to pay extra attention to your posture, making more effort to stretch and strengthen your shoulders and back.

For instance, as a woman with boobs, it is absolutely excruciating for me to do any posture in which I have to lie on my belly with my hands beside my hips. (The same is true when I'm having a massage.) So I make an adjustment and move my hands up, keeping my arms bent, until they're just under my shoulders, to take the weight. To find an adjustment that works for you, try also keeping your arms straight but tucking them under your hipbones, between your hips and the mat, which also eases some of the pressure.

The absolute biggest challenge with boobs is Shoulderstand (see page 116). There they are, literally in your face, compressing your lungs. This is the reason I tend to keep Shoulderstand short, and focus on keeping my breath deep and rhythmically even; otherwise I can feel as if I'm drowning or suffocating. So my advice is: never feel shy about adjusting a position a little if you're uncomfortable. And reassure yourself that human nature being what it is, flatter-chested women in the class are probably sneaking an envious peek, wishing they had such problems.

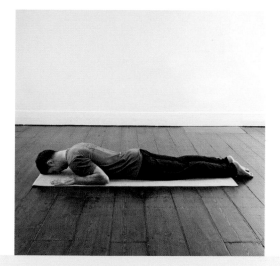

Backbends can't be rushed: you need to get the body used to them, because it's such an unfamiliar position in our forward-hunched lives

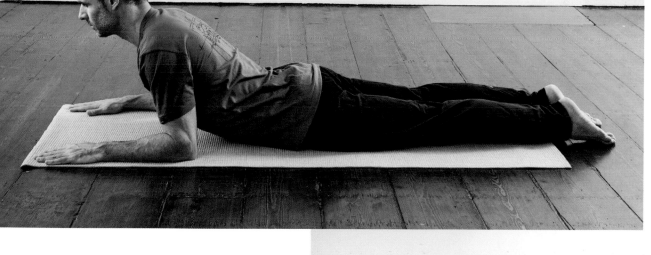

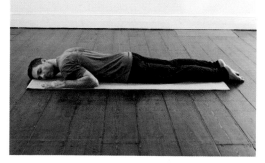

Bridge Pose (Setu Bandha Sarvangasana)
BACKBENDING: MEDIUM DIFFICULTY

Those who follow the philosophical side of yoga say that Bridge Pose helps to unite the physical self with the spiritual self. It is also a good pose with which to start exploring backbends in a safe and gentle way. This version is a gradual easing into Bridge Pose, and avoids any strain that can result from going straight into 'full' bridge. I've always found this insight from one of my yoga teachers hugely helpful: when you're lowering the spine to the ground, imaging you're placing a sleeping baby on the ground. Yes, truly, you need to be that gentle!

GOOD FOR:
- **Strengthening the abdominal and pelvic-floor muscles**
- **Boosting leg strength**
- **Stimulating the spine and the lymph glands in the neck**

START BY: lying flat on your back, with your arms alongside your body. Bend both knees and bring your heels as close to your buttocks as you comfortably can, keeping your feet hip-width apart and flat on the mat.

1 On an out-breath and using your arms for support, gently raise your buttocks off the mat just a few centimetres. Don't clench the muscles in your backside; just hang there for a few breaths.

2 Very slowly, vertebra by vertebra, lower your spine on an out-breath, until your bottom is back on the mat.

3 On another out-breath, lift your hips off the floor again, this time to the point at which your mid-back lifts off the mat. Again, just hang there, buttocks released, and breathe.

4 Once again, lower your bottom to the mat, vertebra by vertebra and on an out-breath.

Variation I
I like to practise Bridge Pose using a prop: a brick-shaped cork block or solid rectangular foam block, placed on its end. I place it in the curve of my lower back once I'm up in the final position. With this support it's easier to relax and get the full benefit of the spinal stretch. Place the block within easy reach before going up into bridge so that you don't have to look to slip it into place.

Variation II
Once you're resting on your shoulders, lift your arms over your head, and rest them on the floor behind you. While in this position, you can also raise your heels off the floor, either one at a time or both together. This slightly advanced variation is quite easily done after a little regular practice.

5 Now you've loosened up your spine, you're ready for 'full' bridge. On an out-breath, really draw up your abdominal, and pelvic muscles, using this energy to lift your hips off the floor. This time, aim to lift your back off the floor to shoulder level, or as near as you can get.

6 Keep your arms strong and straight on either side of your body to support the lift. If you're more advanced, clasp your hands together on the floor directly under your back and straighten your arms. Alternatively, lift your hands, with your arms bent at the elbow, and place them under the arch of your lower back if you find the support helpful.

7 Once you're in position, pull your shoulder blades together and see if you can lift a little further. Consciously open your chest while you do this. Hold the position for a few breaths initially; as you grow stronger, you can maintain this posture for longer.

8 Place your arms on the floor beside you; once again, lower your spine vertebra by vertebra until your bottom is back on the mat.

Do...
- Remember to breathe!

Don't...
- Allow your knees to bow out; your legs should stay aligned and your feet parallel and firmly rooted.
- Lift your head from the ground, which will strain your neck.

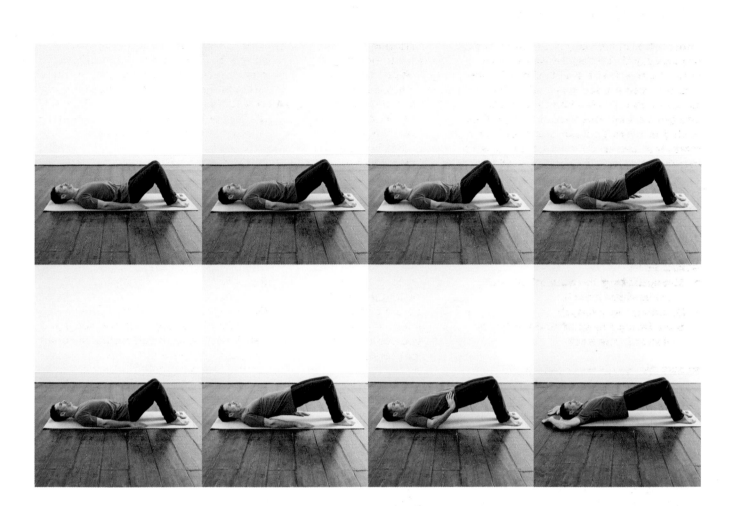

Those who follow the philosophical side of yoga say that Bridge Pose helps to unite the physical self with the spiritual self

Cobra Pose (Bhujangasana)
BACKBENDING: MORE ADVANCED

Since this is called 'Cobra', try to move slowly and gracefully but energetically, like a snake charmer's cobra. It can help – unless you're snake-phobic – to carry that image in your mind. The gentle pressure on the abdominal zone in this pose helps to massage the digestive and reproductive organs, but it's quite a 'warming' posture so don't be surprised if you feel your heat levels rise as you practise. To get used to this type of upper body lift or extension, start by practising Sphinx Pose (see page 90).

GOOD FOR:
- **Strengthening and toning the back muscles**
- **Spinal flexibility**
- **Boosting blood flow**
- **Relieving gynaecological problems**

START BY: lying on your front on the mat, with your legs and abdomen relaxed and your head turned to one side, resting on your hands.

1 Bring your legs together. Turn your head back to centre, resting your forehead on the mat, and slide your arms back so that your hands are in line with your breastbone, fingers pointing forwards. Hug your elbows into your body.

2 As you inhale, slowly raise your forehead so that your nose grazes your mat, then roll your head slightly back so that your chin then brushes the mat.

3 Slowly roll your upper body upwards and backwards. Only rise up as far as is comfortable; ultimately, you may work towards lifting your whole torso off the floor. Keep your arms slightly bent. Over time, work up to staying in this position for up to 30 seconds, but at the beginning aim for ten seconds or so.

4 To come down, slowly lower yourself back onto the mat from the base of your spine, keeping your head tipped very slightly back until you've reached the starting position. Rest your head on the opposite side to the position you began in to rest, then repeat the lift. Build up to four or six lifts altogether.

Do...
- Start with Sphinx Pose (see page 90), and get the hang of that before 'graduating' to Cobra.
- Listen to your lower spine; if you feel a pinching sensation or any form of pain in your lower back as you lift your upper back, come back down and release by going into Child Pose (see page 118).

Don't...
- Use your arms to push up forcibly into Cobra; try to roll the body up into the posture using your torso.
- Lock your elbows and tense your shoulders; these should stay relaxed and down.
- Lift your abdomen off the ground. (Don't get confused with Upward-facing Dog Pose on page 98.)
- Tip your head back too far.

The gentle pressure on the abdominal zone in this pose helps to massage the digestive and reproductive organs

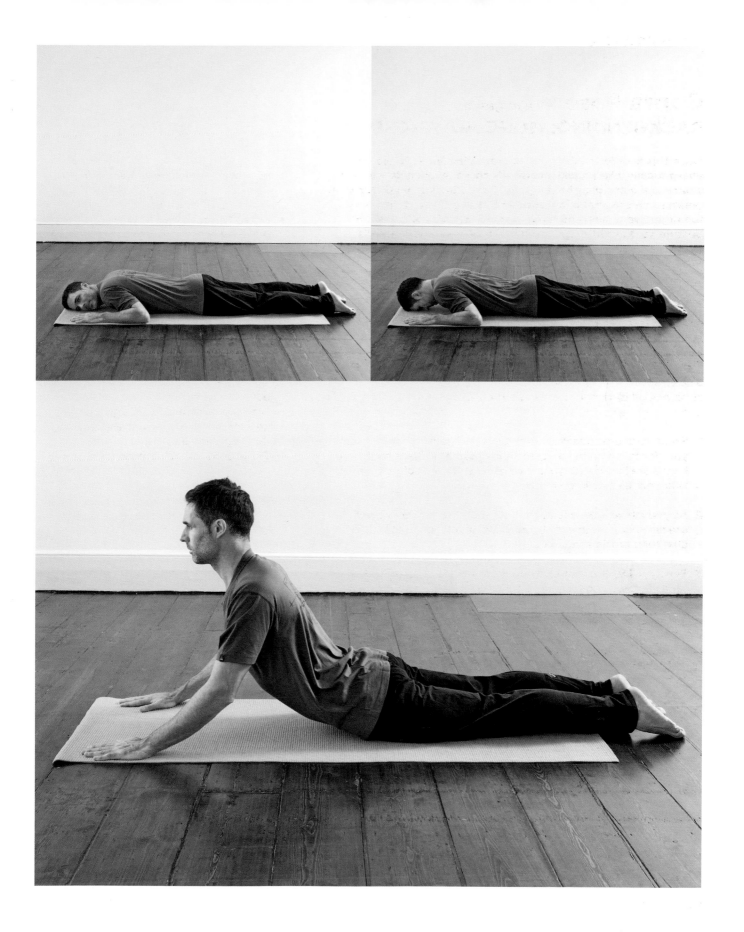

Pigeon Pose (Kapotasana)
BACKBENDING: MORE ADVANCED

Be incredibly cautious when practising this pose if you have previous knee injuries. Of all the postures in this book, this one probably puts most strain on the knee joint.

GOOD FOR:
- **Improving flexibility in the hip joints**
- **Stretching the tight muscles of the backside**

START BY: kneeling on all fours in 'table' position: with your hands under your shoulders and your knees directly under your hips.

1 Bring your right knee forwards and slide your right foot across your left leg, so that the top of the foot and right shin rest on the floor. The further forwards your foot is, the more it pulls on the knee, so don't be ambitious: proceed with caution.

2 Slide your left leg back so that it is straight behind you, with your shin and the top of the left foot resting on the mat. Draw up your pelvic floor and pull your lower abdominal muscles towards your spine.

3 Raise your torso so that you're supporting your weight on your wrists. Again, remain here for just a few seconds to begin with. As the pose becomes more comfortable, stay upright for longer, but be sure to keep your chest up, and to straighten your arms as much as possible without 'locking' them.

4 Lower your upper body so that you rest on your elbows (like Sphinx Pose, see page 90). Breathe deeply and rhythmically. When you begin to practise this pose, stay here for just a few seconds. As you develop your ability to 'rest' into the pose, you can lay your head on your hands on the floor in front of you.

Pigeon is fantastic for improving flexibility in the hip joints

5 Tuck your left foot under and push back into Downward-facing Dog Pose (see page 64), replacing your right foot on the floor, a hip-width's distance from the left foot.

6 Do a 'stepping Dog', a few times: raise one heel so that you stand on the ball of that foot with the other flat on the ground, and then alternate this action between the two feet.

7 Now bring your left leg up to your chest and slide it across your body, lowering your body so that the left leg is angled across you. Follow the steps to repeat the pose on the other side.

Do...
- Only go as far as your knees will allow; if there's any sharp pain at all, come out of the posture straight away, without jerking.
- Try a different, easy way of getting into this posture from Downward Dog: bend one knee to your chest and move the foot across your body until your lower leg is at almost a 90-degree angle, then ease yourself down into Pigeon.

Don't...
- Let your hips get out of alignment. It's easy to twist the hips so that one is further forward, but keep them square to the front of the mat. To get properly aligned, place a folded blanket under your buttock on the side of the front leg if it doesn't touch the mat. This helps to keep your hips square.

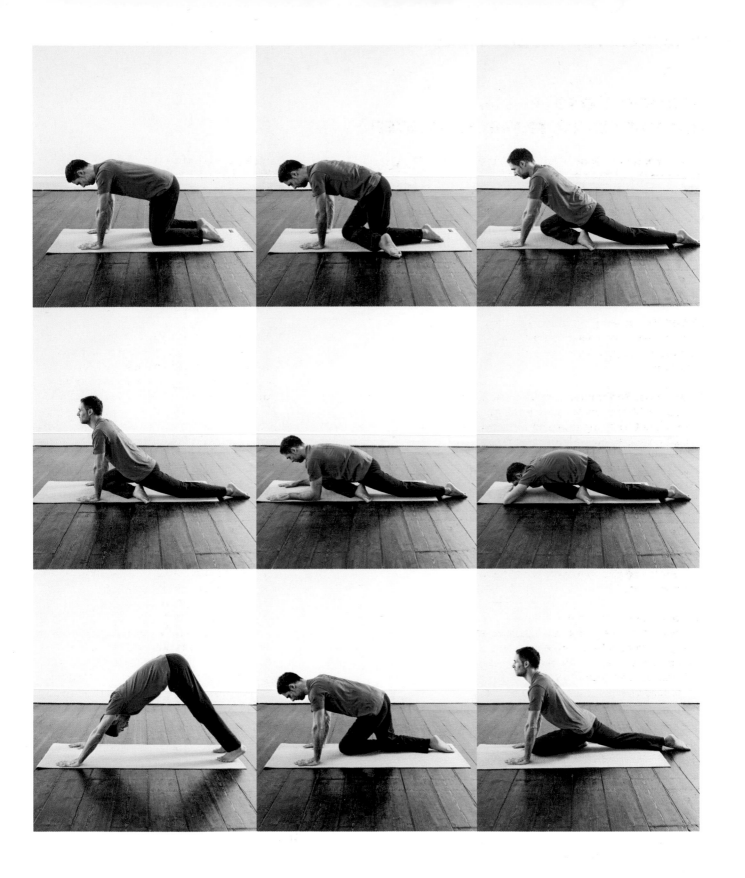

Upward-facing Dog Pose (Urdhva Mukha Svanasana)
BACKBENDING: MORE ADVANCED

This is similar to Cobra Pose (see page 94), but slightly more advanced because you need to have developed the strength to lift your knees off the floor. With regular practice you may eventually progress so that you can begin the posture with your wrists by your waist (an advanced version of this pose).

GOOD FOR:
- **Strengthening the arms, wrists and spine**
- **Relieving mild depression and fatigue**
- **Stretching the chest, shoulders and abdomen**
- **Stimulating digestion**

START BY: lying flat on your mat, face down, with your legs stretched behind you and slightly apart, and the tops of your feet on the mat.

1 Spread your hands and place them beside your shoulders. Press down to straighten your arms; the elbow crease may face slightly forwards.

2 Inhaling, lift your torso upwards and, at the same time, lift your thighs and knees slightly off the floor.

3 Lift your breastbone so that you are looking straight ahead. Draw your shoulders down, away from your ears.

4 Hold the lift for just a few seconds to start with, and gently lower yourself to the mat again, resting your head sideways on the mat. As you become more confident in the pose, add a couple of seconds to the 'hold' each time.

5 Repeat the steps and when you return to the mat, turn your head to the other side to rest.

Do...
- Fold your mat back so that your wrists have extra support, or put a couple of blocks beneath each hand when you begin this exercise if you find it challenging.
- Keep your neck long.

Don't...
- Look upwards, which will compress the neck; look straight ahead.
- Clench the buttocks; they should be 'engaged', but not hard.
- Do this if you have a history of back problems, or RSI/carpal tunnel syndrome. It is also best to avoid it if you have a headache.

This is similar to Cobra Pose, but slightly more advanced because you need to have developed the strength to lift your knees off the floor

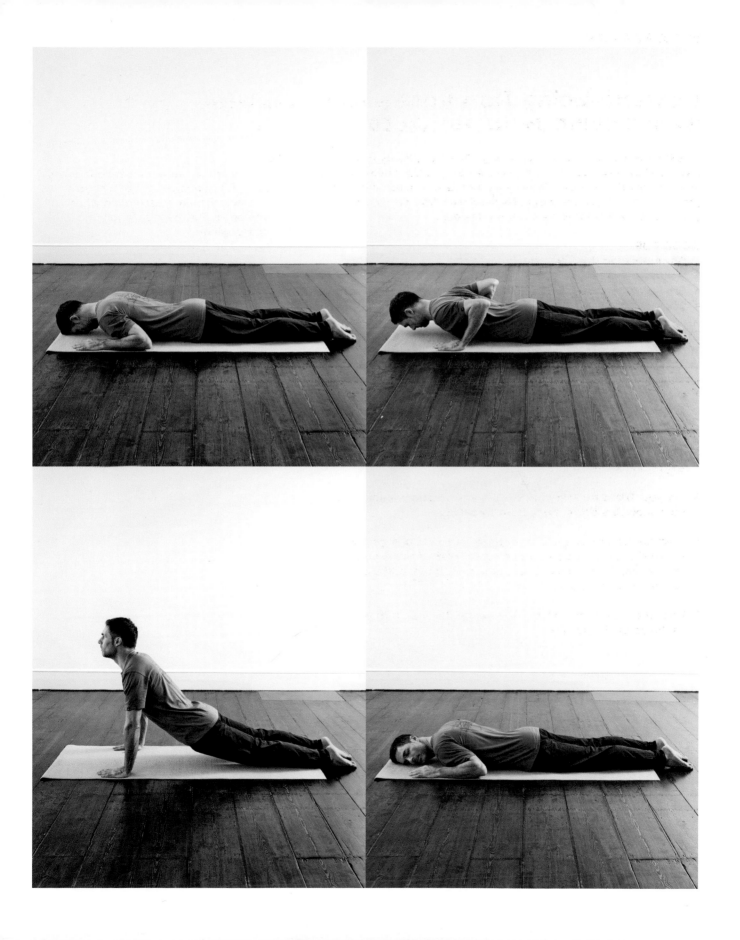

Simple Twist (Bharadvajasana)
TWISTING: BASIC

Literally the simplest and gentlest of twists; if you've never done any yoga before, start with this twist. But this downright feels good any time; like so many postures in the book, it's a fantastic antidote to being seated at a desk, and once you've tried it on the mat, is easy to adapt so that you can do it sitting at an office chair. NB Seek the guidance of an experienced yoga instructor before attempting any kind of twist if you have any lower back or sacroiliac issues.

GOOD FOR:
- **Releasing tension in the mid- and upper back**
- **Massaging the abdominal organs**
- **Enhancing digestion**
- **Strengthening the lower back**
- **Helping to relieve carpal tunnel syndrome and RSI**

START BY: sitting on your mat with your legs straight out in front of you – this is known as Staff Pose (see page 112).

1 Shift onto your right buttock and bend your knees to the opposite side. Rest your feet on the floor, keeping your heels as close to your buttocks as possible. Your left ankle should rest in the arch of your right foot.

2 Breathe in and lift through the front of your body.

3 Breathe out and twist your torso to the right. Keep your left buttock rooted to the ground – when you feel this buttock lifting off, that's as far as you should go. Keep your tummy soft.

4 Place the palm of your left hand on top of your right knee, using it like a lever to get a little more twist. Place your right hand on the floor beside your right buttock – you may have to stretch your fingertips to do this.

Like so many postures in the book, this is a fantastic antidote to being seated at a desk. Once you've tried it on the mat, it is easy to adapt so that you can do it sitting at an office chair

5 Pull your shoulder blades together to open your chest.

6 There are two possible positions for the head; try them both. First, continue the spiral by looking over your right shoulder, staying within the range that is comfortable for your neck. Second, use a 'counter' movement, turning your head so that you are looking over your left shoulder at your feet.

7 As you inhale, continue to lift up through your upper chest and every time you exhale, twist a little further – as far as is comfortable. Hold the twist for 30 seconds to start with, building up to one minute.

8 Release the twist with an out-breath, return to the starting position and repeat the steps to twist to the left, maintaining the hold for the same amount of time. Exit the pose by moving your legs back to the starting position, Staff Pose.

Do...
- Be careful (especially when getting up) if you have high or low blood pressure.
- Be conscious of sinking both 'sitting bones' into the ground. To help this, place a folded blanket under the buttock you're leading the twist with. (That's the right buttock, if you follow the instructions above. When you switch sides, move the blanket so it's positioned under the left buttock.)

Don't...
- Do this twist before bedtime, since it can be stimulating.
- Tilt towards the twisting side. Use the blanket trick, above, if this happens.

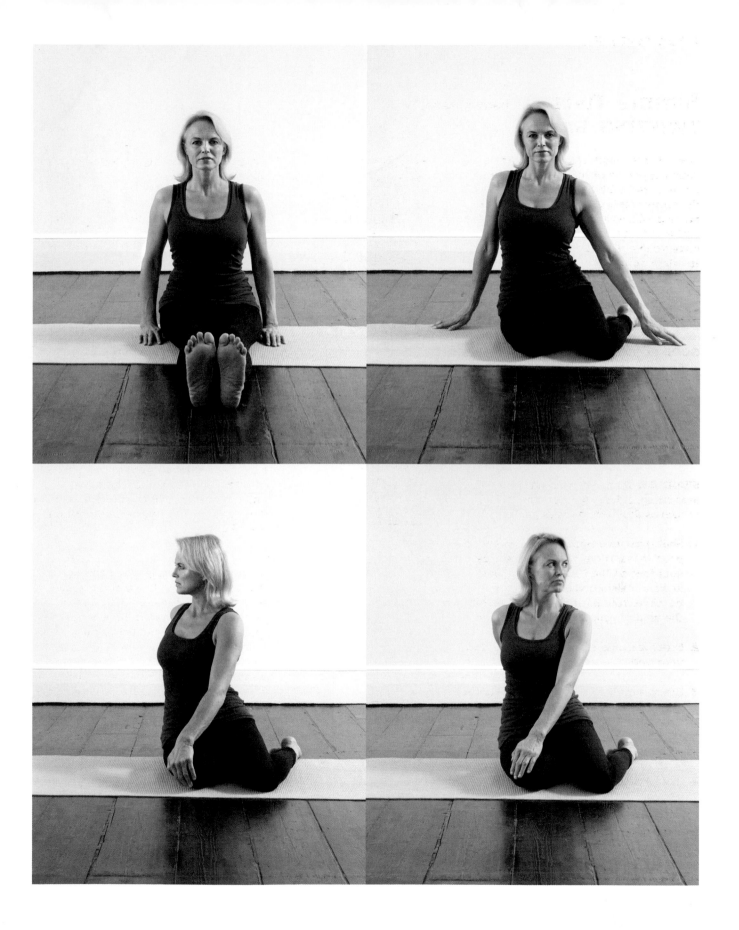

Chair Twist variation
TWISTING: BASIC

**For an even simpler twist, you just need a dining chair.
This is a valuable twist for elderly people who tend to lose
mobility in the spine; it can be done very, very gently.**

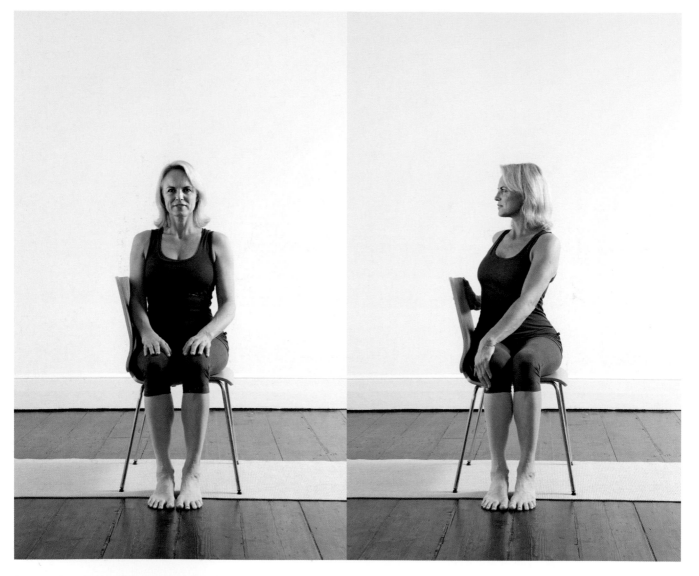

1 Start by sitting sideways on the chair,
with the back of the chair positioned to
your right. Bring your knees together
and make sure your feet are firmly on
the floor, heels directly below your
knees.

2 Exhale and twist towards the back of the
chair, placing the palm of your left hand
on the outside of your right knee. Stay
here for a few seconds.

Use a chair that's the right height for your feet to comfortably rest flat on the floor

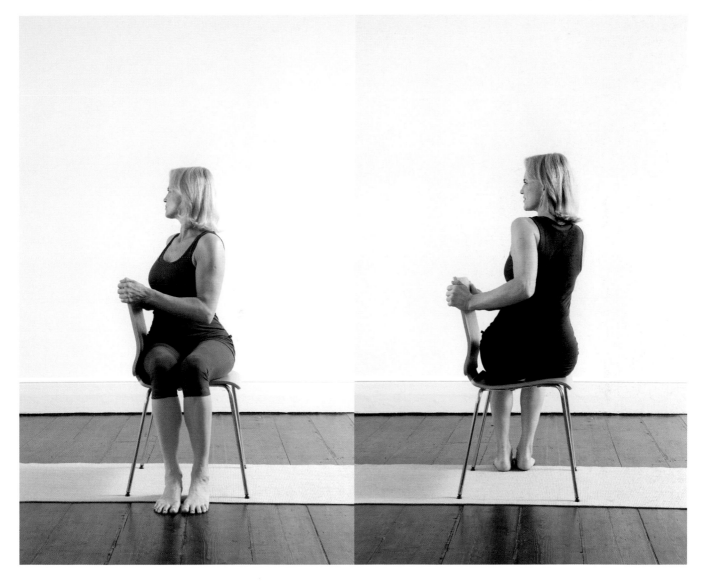

3 Lift both hands and place them on either side of the chair-back, then push your palms together slightly: this will give your shoulder blades a good stretch. Hold the twist for 30 seconds.

4 Return to your starting position and then move to the other side of the chair, with the back positioned to your left. Repeat the instructions to twist in the other direction.

Two-legged Reclining Twist
TWISTING: BASIC

Reclining twists are the perfect final postures in a yoga sequence, preparing you for relaxation. (I also find them fantastic first thing in the morning for relieving stiffness, making my spine feel flowing and free – and also very useful after a long walk, which can be a bit punishing on the hips.) It feels fantastic to 'wring out' the body in this way.

GOOD FOR:
- **Sluggish digestion**
- **Back and neck tension**
- **Soothing frazzled nerves**
- **Boosting energy**
- **Improving breathing**

START BY: lying flat on your back on the mat.

1 Bend your knees and place your feet slightly apart on your mat, with the soles of your feet roughly 30cm away from your tailbone.

2 Rest your arms straight out beside you, palms facing upwards at shoulder level. Let your shoulders sink into the floor.

3 As you exhale, slowly drop your knees to the left, maintaining contact between the edge of your left foot and the floor. Your knees may not reach anywhere near the floor; that's fine.

I find reclining twists fantastic first thing in the morning for relieving stiffness, making my spine feel flowing and free – and also very useful after a long walk, which can be a bit punishing on the hips

4 Press down firmly through your right shoulder to ensure that you have contact with the floor. (It's important that the shoulder doesn't lift up from the ground.) Turn your head towards the right.

5 Stay in the pose for four or five deep, long breaths. Then lift your knees back to their starting position and repeat on the other side.

Do...
- Use this as a gentle introduction to the different reclining twists, rather than going straight for the intensive version – your body will thank you...
- Let gravity do the work.

Don't...
- Force your legs towards the mat; let them go as far as is comfortable. This will soon improve.
- Lift the opposite shoulder off the mat; it's more important to keep this shoulder grounded than to drop your legs further to the opposite side.
- Strain your neck; only turn your head as far as is entirely comfortable.

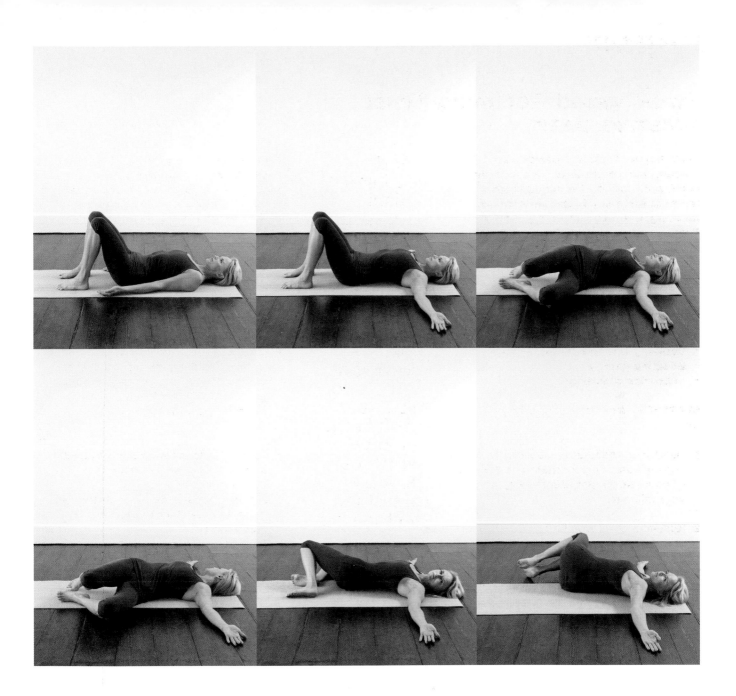

More Intense Reclining Twist
TWISTING: MEDIUM DIFFICULTY

Instead of twisting from the hips, you're really twisting from the waist in this version. This is slightly more advanced but after you've mastered the simple reclining twist you should be able to progress swiftly to this – which (as postures go) most students find pretty addictive, in my experience.

GOOD FOR:
All the same reasons as the previous twist, but also excellent for **stretching out the lower back and sacroiliac joint**, and for **toning the waist area**.

START BY: lying flat on your back on the mat with your knees bent and feet flat on the floor.

1 Lift your knees towards your chest, then extend your arms at shoulder height, palms facing upwards. The higher you draw your knees before twisting, the more challenging this pose becomes.

2 Lower your knees to the left very slowly and in a controlled way.

3 When your knees reach the mat, place your left hand on top of your thigh, and press down to anchor yourself in the pose. It's important that your legs are really resting on the ground. Turn your head to face right.

4 Stay here for four or five long breaths (extending this as you become more practised). Draw in your abdominal muscles and lift your bent legs back towards your chest. Bring your head back to the centre, too.

5 Gradually lower your knees to the right and repeat to the other side, moving your head to face left.

Do...
• Keep your back long and straight on the mat.
• Place a small folded blanket under your head, if this feels more comfortable.

Don't...
• Raise your knees up so high if your legs don't easily reach the ground when you twist.
• Strain as you look over the shoulder opposite the legs; only turn your head as far as is comfortable.
• Try this is you have lower back injuries or a herniated disc, or if you are pregnant.

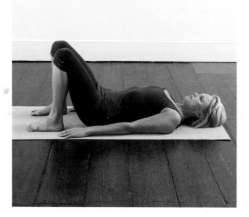

This twist is excellent for stretching out the lower back and sacroiliac joint, and for toning the waist area

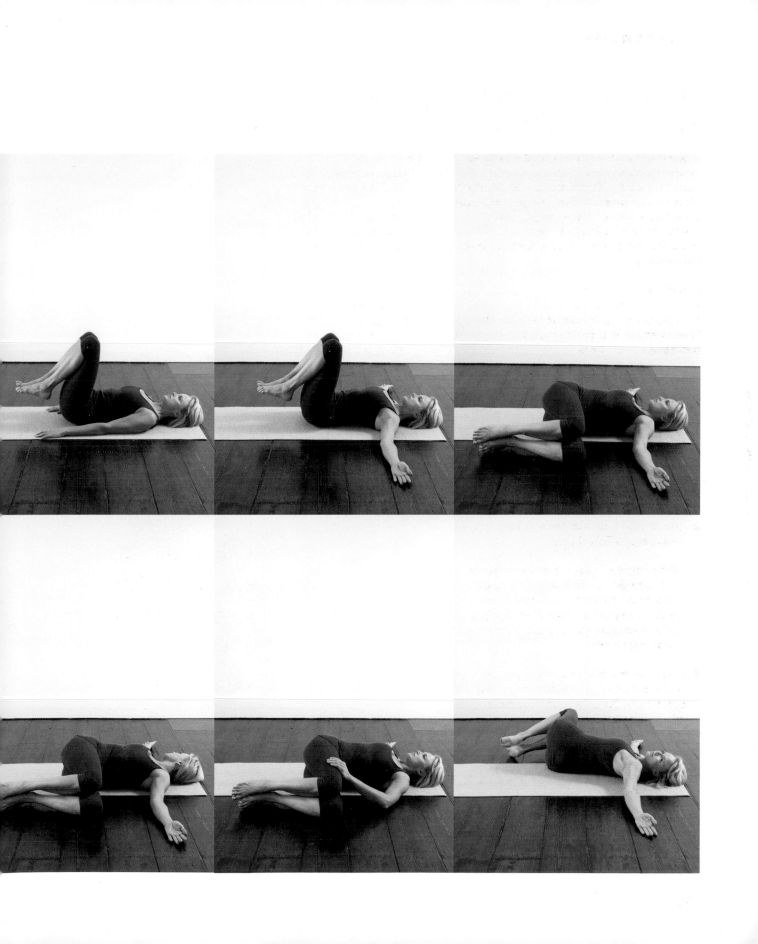

Supported Reclining Twist
TWISTING: MEDIUM DIFFICULTY

Since it soothes frazzled nerves while boosting energy, I find this is a great pose to do on the office floor! In Yin or Restorative yoga classes (see pages 34–5), you might stay in this pose for five or ten minutes, believe it or not, but when you're beginning to learn it, just surrender to it for a few seconds.

Good for:
- **Improving breathing**
- **Easing everyday tension in the back and neck**
- **Boosting hip flexibility**
- **Enhancing digestion**

START BY: placing a bolster or a couple of cushions at hip-height on the left side of your body. You may also want to place a 'squishy block' or a cushion beneath your head. Then lie on your back on the mat, with your legs bent and your feet resting on the floor.

1 Lengthen your spine as much as you can by lifting your hips off the ground and drawing your tailbone towards your heels, then place your hips back down on the mat. Relax here for a few moments.

2 Bring your right knee towards you and, using your right hand, grab the back of your right thigh, or your shin. Rock from side to side a little, to massage your lower back, and start to breathe more slowly and deeply.

3 Slowly straighten the opposite leg towards the end of your mat (in this case, your left leg). Stretch your arms out at shoulder height.

4 Roll your right leg over your left leg, while keeping the straight leg more or less in place. At the same time, roll your torso and both arms over to your left side, arcing the top arm until one palm is stacked on top of the other (it's almost like rolling over in bed).

Do...
- Make sure you get your props in place before you start.
- Feel like you're sinking into the earth.
- Relax into Corpse Pose (see pages 132–4) after this pose.

Don't...
- Allow the opposite shoulder to your twisted leg to lift off the floor.

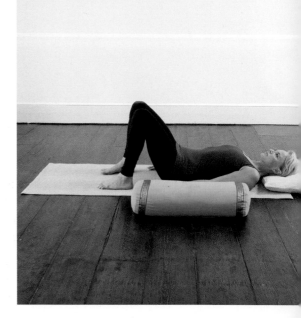

Your knee should come to rest on the bolster or cushions, which should offer enough support that you can simply sink all your weight into them. Soften your body, feel your skin relax and surrender to the stretch for 30–60 seconds at the beginning. Lengthen the time you hold the pose as it becomes more comfortable.

5 Now comes the full twist. 'Arc' your right arm up and over to the right-hand side of your body, stretching it out at shoulder height and following it with your gaze. Stay here for 30–60 seconds to start with, building up the time you can rest into the position each time you practise.

6 Then roll your right leg back to the centre, bring your extended leg towards your chest and give yourself a hug, before moving the bolster or cushions to the other side and repeating on the opposite side.

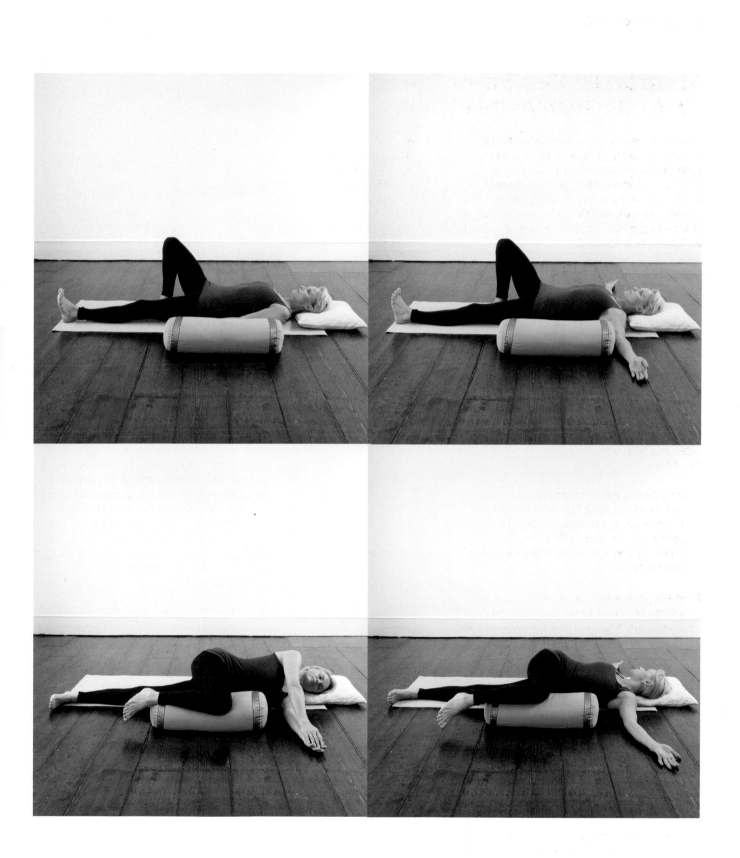

Easy Pose (Sukhasana)
SITTING: BASIC

This is an ideal position for meditation since it allows energy to flow freely through the body and (after a bit of practice) can be maintained for quite some time. It is the 'easy' version of Lotus Pose (Padmasana) (in which the legs are crossed tight to the body, and the feet tucked above either knee), which can be dodgy for older knees, unless you have a lot of yoga experience. I would not advise anyone to try Lotus Pose except under the supervision of a teacher. Happily, Easy Pose shares many of the benefits of Lotus. But don't be deceived by the name: most of us spend a lot of time sitting in chairs, and crossing the legs in this way is unfamiliar to us as adults – challenging, even. Easy Pose should be practised with especial caution if you have any kind of knee problem. Never go further than is comfortable.

GOOD FOR:
- **Learning how to sit comfortably as a preparation for meditation**
- **Calming the mind**
- **Strengthening the back, both spine and muscles**

START BY: folding a blanket (or two) to make a square support about 15cm in height. Sit on the edge of the support, with your 'sitting bones' on the blanket and your legs stretched out in front of you on the mat, in Staff Pose (see page 112). Alternatively, rest your backside on a firm bolster.

> Most of us spend a lot of time sitting in chairs but this stretches the hips – and allows energy to flow freely

1 Fold your legs in towards your body, crossing your knees and slipping each foot beneath the opposite knee.

2 Make sure your feet are relaxed and that there is a comfortable gap between your pelvis and your feet.

3 Breathe easily and start to relax your mind. Start by holding for a minute, and build up from there until you can comfortably hold the pose for several minutes; you may want to reverse the leg positions so the opposite knee is on top, to feel physically 'balanced'.

4 To get out of the pose, carefully straighten your legs into Staff Pose again.

Do...
- Feel 'grounded' through your hips and legs.
- Gently lean your torso forwards, after you have become used to this pose over time; this gives a great stretch to the buttocks. Only lean as far forwards as is comfortable, though; don't put extra pressure on the knees.

Don't...
- Let your back slump or tuck your pelvis so that your weight rests on your tailbone. Keep your spine upright. (Use that trick of imagining there's a thread lifting up the top of your head.)
- Don't over-arch your back and stick your chest out. You should be sitting beautifully straight, not sagging front or back.

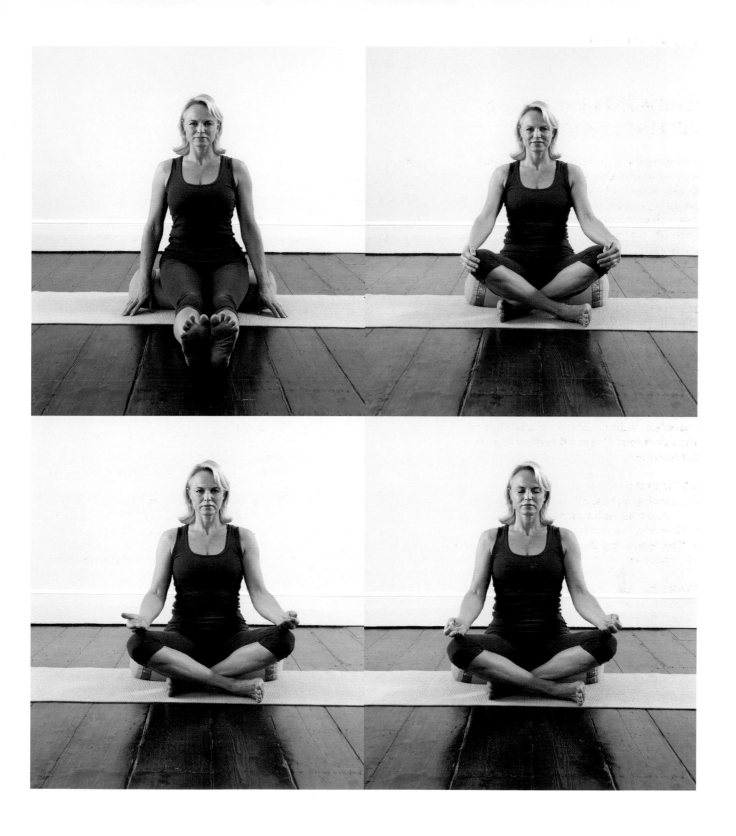

Staff Pose (Dandasana)
SITTING: BASIC

Be aware of your posture in this pose; you should feel as if the crown of your head is being lifted by a string. If you're not sure whether you are properly aligned, practise the pose with your buttocks and shoulders pressing against a wall.

GOOD FOR:
• **Strengthening the back muscles**
• **Targeting 'bingo wings'**
• **Improving posture**

START BY: sitting on the mat with your legs together and straight out in front of you. Place your feet together, toes pointing upwards. Place your hands directly below your shoulders, beside your hips on the floor – with your fingers pointing forwards. Position a folded blanket under your sitting bones if you feel as if you're tilting back. This shifts the pelvis forwards a little.

1 Firm your thighs and feel them pressing down into the mat (or the folded blanket if you are using one), and rotate them inwards slightly.

2 Flex your ankles and press out through your heels and the balls of your feet, so your feet are 'firm' and your toes are pointing slightly back towards you.

3 Imagine energy is streaming upwards through your torso, up over your head and down your back into the floor. Feel your spine lengthening as you visualise this.

4 Think of your spine as a 'staff' right in the middle of your upright body as you hold the pose for a minute or so. Then relax.

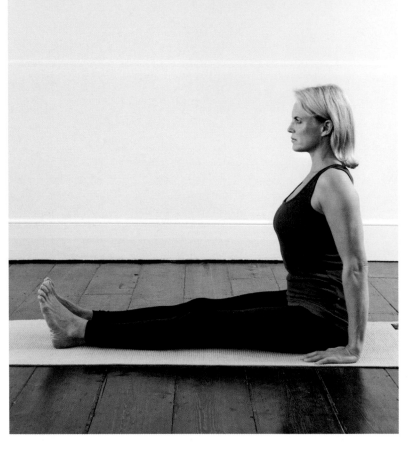

In this pose you should feel as if the crown of your head is being lifted by a string

Do...
• Place a couple of bricks or blocks on either side of your thighs, if you have a long back – which may mean your arms don't reach the ground (mine don't). These should be the right height to allow you to straighten your back fully, but not to 'lift' you off the ground.

Don't...
• Stay too long in the pose if you have wrist weakness or problems.

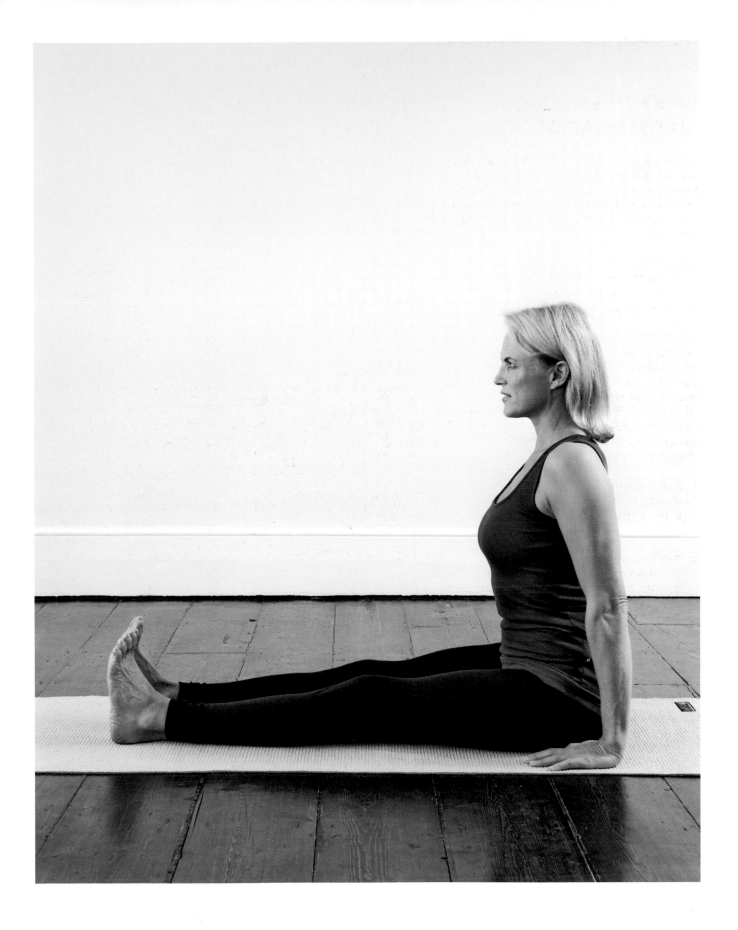

Legs-up-the-wall Pose (Viparita Karani)
INVERSION: BASIC

This is a brilliant alternative to a headstand or shoulderstand since although it is an 'inversion' (allowing blood to flow back to the heart and brain), it does not put the same amount of stress on the shoulders, neck or head as those postures do. If I only have 30 minutes to revive myself after a hard day at work before a party, I'll spend 15 of them doing this. It's also a fantastic pose to practise before bed if you have trouble sleeping.

GOOD FOR:
- **Promoting restful sleep**
- **Relieving tired legs**

START BY: folding a firm woollen blanket into a rectangular shape approximately 30cm x 60cm. Place this 'support' 20–30cm away from a bare wall (it's best to practise this pose in a space free from furniture or pictures). Place another further down the mat for your head to rest on.

1 Sit on the folded blanket with your legs parallel to the wall, and bend your knees.

2 Shift your position so that you bring your lower back onto the floor and swing your legs up the wall. Use your elbows to support you as you lower your back onto the ground. When you're in position, your back will be at a 90-degree angle to the wall.

3 Roll your shoulders backwards to open your chest, and rest your arms alongside your torso.

4 Feel your spine and the whole of your back sinking into the ground. Breathe deeply and slowly, and with each breath feel your tension melting away and your heart opening.

> If I only have 30 minutes to revive myself after a hard day at work before a party, I'll spend 15 of them doing this

5 If you're comfortable in the position, rest here for several minutes.

6 To deepen the posture, raise your arms and place them behind your head, resting them on the ground, slightly bent at the elbow or crossing at the wrists. If this is too much of a stretch, place two cushions just behind you, where your elbows bend, and rest your arms on these. (Get these into place before going into the pose.)

7 To come out bring your knees into your chest and roll onto your side. Stay for a breath or two before pushing yourself into an upright position.

Do...
- Shuffle to get your bottom as close to the wall as possible.
- Stay for as long as you like in the pose, especially if you have weary legs.
- Bend at the knees to rest the soles of your feet on the wall, rather than the backs of your thighs, if the leg stretch is too extreme for you.
- Place an eye pillow on your eyelids, for even greater relaxation.
- Progress to using a bolster instead of a folded blanket – this arches the spine more. Place the bolster away from the wall, so it's underneath your middle back, then do a bit of 'schnoofling' around to make sure you're in the right position. You'll soon learn the perfect distance for your anatomy.

Don't...
- Use a bolster (see above) if you have back problems, since it can over-arch a troubled back.

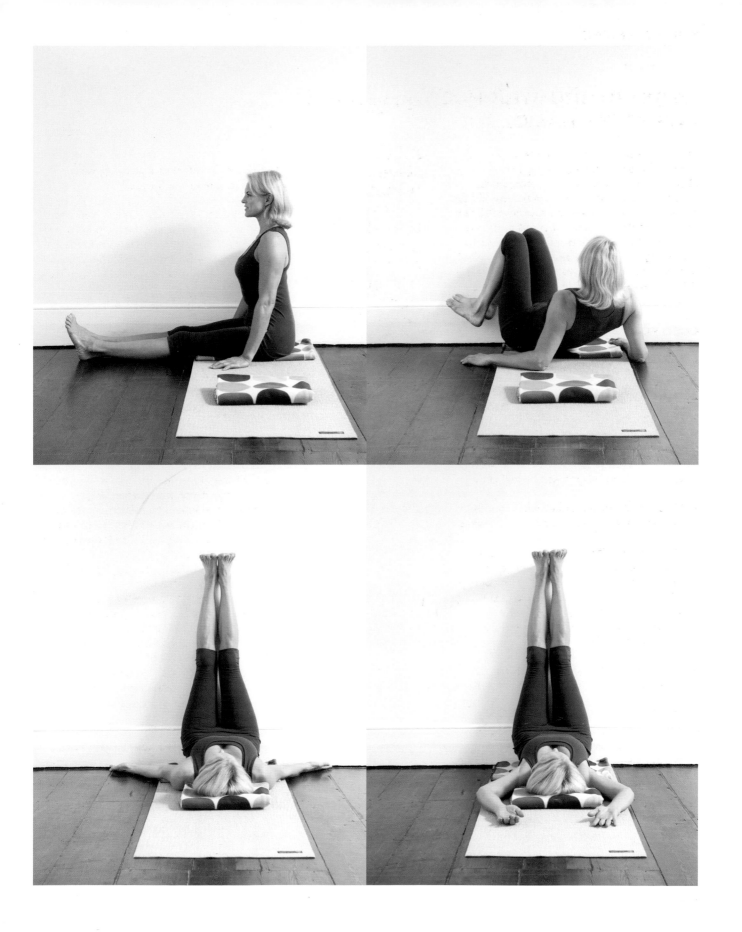

Supported Shoulderstand (Salamba Sarvangasana)
INVERSION: ADVANCED

This supported version of the hugely beneficial Shoulderstand is easier for beginners than the classical pose taught in many classes because it is practised next to a wall, for security. When you start practising, I suggest you place the pile of blankets about 30cm away from the wall, and use the wall to help 'lever' yourself into position. As you become comfortable with the pose, you may no longer need the wall, but if you'd like to move towards an unsupported Shoulderstand, do this under the supervision of a qualified yoga teacher before attempting it at home.

GOOD FOR:
- **Calming the brain**
- **Stimulating the thyroid and parathyroid glands**, located in the neck
- **Benefiting the abdominal organs, and the prostate (in men)**
- **Relieving menopausal symptoms**
- **Beating fatigue and helping with insomnia**

START BY: placing your yoga mat with the thin end against a wall (make sure the wall is free from furniture or pictures). Fold a firm woollen blanket into a rectangular shape, approximately 60cm x 80cm. Place the blanket with the long side parallel to and directly against the wall.

1 Sit sideways beside the pile of blankets, with your legs parallel to the wall. (Experiment a few times with distances to get this right.) The 'goal' position is to have your shoulders, but not your head, resting on the folded blankets, to elevate your neck and prevent strain.

2 As you exhale, swing your shoulders down so they're positioned over the edge of the blanket, as above. At the same time, swing your legs up onto the wall, with your buttocks touching the wall. (At this point, your legs are straight.) You may have to shimmy a bit to get in the right position. Rest your arms alongside your body, palms down.

3 Bend your knees and slide your feet down until you can flatten the soles to the wall. Push your feet into the wall and lift your hips. Make sure you feel completely supported. Squeeze your shoulder blades together, bend your elbows and place your hands underneath your hips so that they fully support the weight of your lower body.

4 Gently 'kick off' with one leg and straighten that leg; if you feel as if you have complete support, remove your second leg from the wall and straighten that one too. Walk your hands 'up' your back a little, more towards your shoulders. Try to keep your elbows as close together as you can.

5 Raise your pelvis so that it's directly over your shoulders, stretching your feet. If you were to draw a line from your feet to your shoulders, it would be straight.

6 Once you are in position, firm up your legs; turn your thighs inwards slightly and, on an inhalation, firm your knees. Don't point your toes ballerina-style, but lift through the ball of each foot and pull the toes very slightly towards your head.

7 The back of your head should now be resting on the floor so that your forehead is parallel to the floor and your chin perpendicular to it. Look at your chest, but keep your gaze soft. Although you may be feeling quite stressed at this point, especially the first few times you practise, consciously soften your throat and tongue.

8 Stay up in the pose for just 15–30 seconds the first time you practise. Add 5–10 more seconds each time you practise. Ultimately, yoga experts advise working towards holding for three minutes, but that could take years. When you're ready to come out of the pose, lower your legs slightly towards your head and move your hands towards your waist (make sure they still support your body fully). Place one foot on the wall, then the other, and slowly replace your spine on the pile of blankets, vertebra by vertebra, until your whole back is resting on the ground.

9 Stretch your legs up the wall, draw your toes gently towards you and gently rest.

10 Finally, lower your legs alongside the wall while levering yourself, using your elbow, into a sitting position.

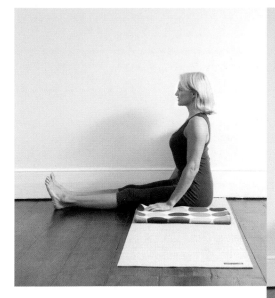

Do...

- Allow yourself a bit of playtime to get the positioning of the blankets and mat right. You may need to go up and come down a few times to get it right, but you'll soon get the hang of it.
- Try to keep your elbows close together rather than allowing them to 'splay'.
- Keep one leg on the wall at first, to help you balance while you get used to the inversion.
- B-R-E-A-T-H-E. Your chin rests on your chest in this pose, which can feel quite stressful and claustrophobic, especially if you have a generous bust, and if you don't make a conscious effort, your breathing can 'freeze'.
- Try the pose away from the wall eventually, once you feel comfortable going up and coming back down. However, I've been doing this pose for years and I still like the 'security-blanket' feeling a wall gives me.

Don't...

- Bend your knees when you're up in the pose; they should remain straight. Don't separate your legs, either.
- 'Crunch' your neck – try to keep it long.
- Freak out about the fact that any excess weight feels like it's cascading down towards you in the pose. It is normal for anyone who's less than completely toned to feel flabby in Shoulderstand. Be aware that the pose does get easier and less stressful.
- Stay too long in the pose, to start with.

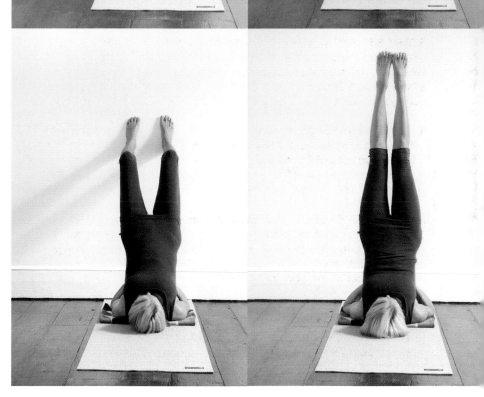

As you become comfortable with shoulderstand, you may eventually find you don't need the wall

Child Pose (Balasana)
RESTING: BASIC

I think of this as the 'default' posture in yoga, because in so many of the gentle classes that I like to do, or at home, it's wonderful to slip into Child Pose to rest the body when it's been exerted, or as a counterposture to Downward Dog, or to backbends. But despite the 'childlike' name, it's not always easy and you may find Wide-Legged Child Pose (pictured) suits you better, or that you benefit from some of the props suggested at the end of the instructions.

GOOD FOR:
- **Stretching the legs, from ankles to thighs and hips**
- **Calming a busy mind**
- **De-stressing**

START BY: kneeling on your mat, mid-way down the mat, facing the front (short end) of the mat.

1 With your toes touching, lean back until you're sitting on your heels.

2 Separate your knees slightly so they're about hip-width apart.

3 Breathe out, then lay your upper body down over your thighs. Gently stretch out your neck as you move towards the floor.

4 Move your hands back alongside your body, palms facing upwards; your hands and arms should feel heavy on the ground. Enjoy the stretch this gives to your shoulder and mid-back. (See 'Do...' right.)

5 Breathe deeply and rhythmically; hold for just 30 seconds, to begin with, and build up to a few minutes.

6 Straighten the front of your torso, lifting your head from the ground; breathe in and lift from the tailbone, until you're sitting upright with your hands beside your sides.

Do...
- Place a bolster or thickly folded blanket between your feet and your bottom, if you have previously had knee problems or you simply find this tough on your knees. It is really important to communicate any knee issues to a teacher, before going into Child Pose in a class for the first time.
- Support the head, if you have neck problems; try placing a small folded blanket under your forehead to support it, or resting your forehead on folded hands.
- Place a folded blanket under your legs – from knee to toe – if you find that the top of your foot feels painful against the mat.
- Sink more deeply into this posture with every breath.
- Stretch your arms forward, in front of you, if resting your forehead on the ground feels in any way uncomfortable. (In my case, a previous whiplash injury makes it impossible to do the 'classic' Child Pose.)
- Try the 'wide-kneed' alternative to Child pose: your toes are touching but your knees are much wider apart than hip-width. This makes it possible to sink your upper body much closer to the floor, resting your forehead either on your folded hands, or stretching the arms in front of you on the mat. Personally? I think this is 'friendlier' to mature bodies...

Don't...
- Go deeply into Child if you have knee problems (see bolster tip, above).

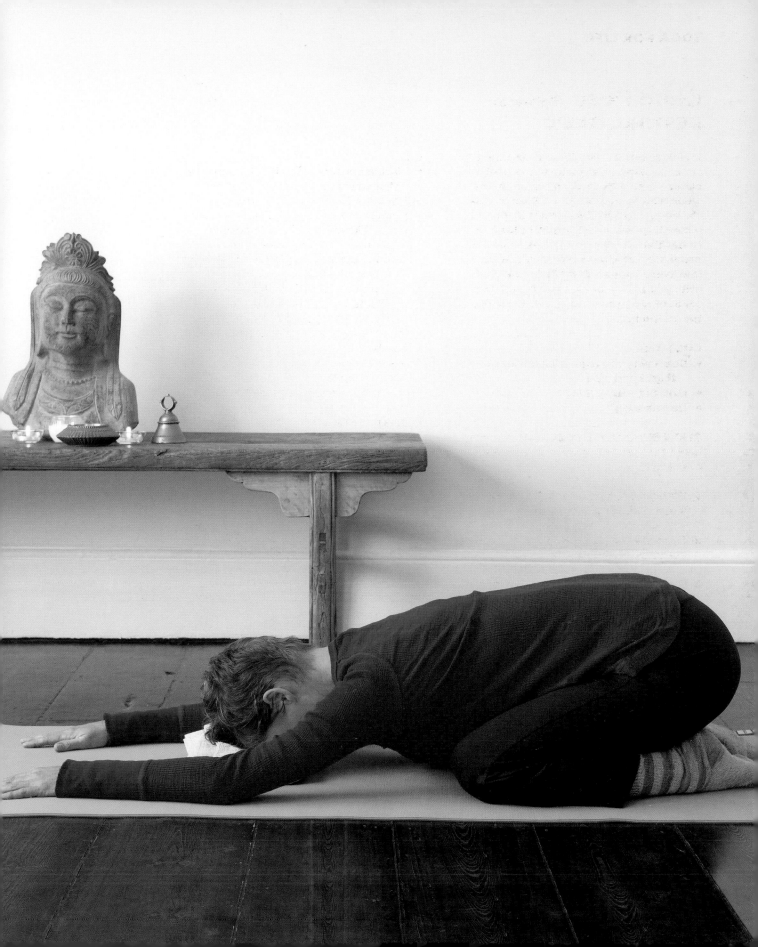

Supported Relaxation Pose
RESTING: BASIC

A yoga session always ends with relaxation in Corpse Pose. Full instructions for this pose are given on pages 132–4, but this is a supported variation. It takes a little longer to set up, but is the ultimate relaxation pose, and it really is worth the extra hassle of gathering the props. Feeling supported in this pose is almost like being cocooned, and it allows you to sink deep into a blissful state of total relaxation.

GOOD FOR:
- **Allowing yourself to sink more deeply into rest**
- **Lowering blood pressure**
- **Easing fatigue**
- **Insomnia and various types of headache (not a universal panacea, but many people find this useful)**

START BY: finding a piece of furniture that's just the right height for your legs to rest on. This might be a stool, a bench, a small side table, or maybe the edge of the sofa with the cushions removed. Scrabble around on your backside to figure out a restful height, then position your mat with the narrow end against the support. Make sure you have everything you'll need in the pose close at hand: a timer, blanket, a small cushion, folded blanket or baby's pillow for your head, and a sandbag and eye pillow if you would like to use one (see page 124). Put on socks if your feet get cold when you lie still.

1 Lie on your back on your mat and swing your legs up to rest on your support. Check that your knees are bent at a perfect 90-degree angle, and that your calves and heels are resting comfortably on the support.

2 Check that your lower back is resting comfortably on the mat, and is not tilted in any way.

3 Support your head with the cushion, folded blanket or pillow, then set your alarm for 15 or (even better) 30 minutes.

It really is worth the extra hassle of gathering the props for this deep relaxation, which is like being cocooned

Place a sandbag on your lower abdomen and an eye pillow over your eyes, if you like the sensation.

4 Now use your breath to drop into the relaxation, following the instructions on page 133.

5 When time's up, slide the sandbag (if using) off your body to the left, bend your knees to your chest and roll onto your right side. An eye pillow will fall off as you roll over, so keep your eyes covered with your fingers for a few seconds, then gradually open them to let light in. Use your arms to push yourself up to a sitting position.

Do...
- Start by practising Legs-up-the-wall Pose (see page 114), a supported inversion, which is also incredibly, blissfully, fabulously relaxing.
- Take the time to find the right props and have them within reach.
- Be sure to wear enough clothes to keep you toasty; it's amazing how quickly the body cools down.

Don't...
- Rest your legs on a too-high piece of furniture, as this isn't good for your back. If you don't have something the right height, just stick with Legs-up-the-wall.

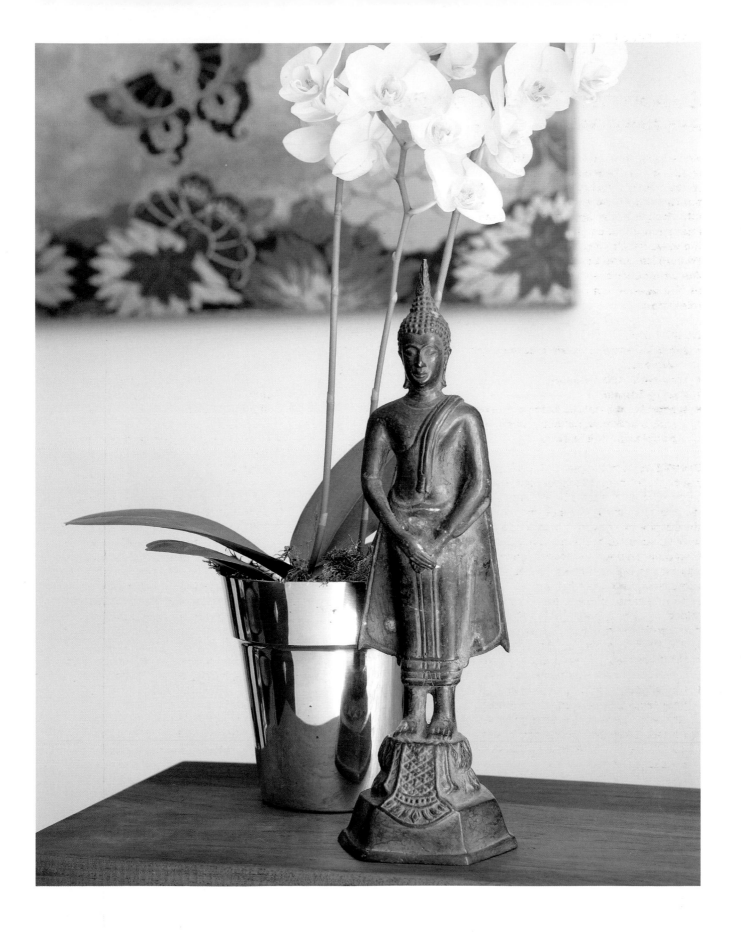

Putting together a sequence

In the step-by-step instructions (see pages 60–120) I have organised the yoga postures by category: Standing, Balancing, Backbending, and so on. To create the perfect sequence, you would ideally choose a posture from each category, starting and finishing with a Resting pose. At the start of your sequence, the Resting posture acts as a form of preparation, allowing you to slough off the angst and pressures you brought to the mat, and to start to integrate body, breath and mind on the mat.

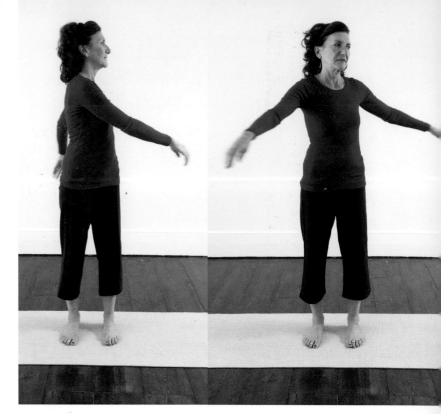

There's a lot of disagreement among yoga practitioners from different traditions (see pages 32–5) about which postures should be done when, and in which order. But there are, in fact, no universal prescriptions. So it's best to think of these postures as like Lego bricks, which can be added one to another as you deepen your practice. There's no need to do them all to start with – after all, you'd never attempt all of them in a single class. A logical, comfortable sequence would follow the pattern in the box on the right, embracing at least one exercise from each 'category'.

In the Yoga Prescriptions chapter (see page 166), you'll also find specific suggestions for sequences of postures that may be helpful with certain challenges – from a headache to menopausal symptoms. Of course there is a big difference between a headache and the menopause; what they have in common is that yoga can help ease either. But whether you are planning a sequence for therapeutic or exercise purposes, there are some basic rules to follow:

How long to allow for a sequence Much depends on how much time you have available. The bottom line is that five minutes is better than no minutes. My recommendation for a home practice is around 10–12 postures, repeating each several times before progressing, seeking each time to go a little 'deeper' into the posture. Above all, don't 'hurry' yoga; go at

> It's best to think of postures like Lego bricks. They can be added one to another as you deepen your practice. There's no need to do them all to start with – you'd never attempt all of them in a single class

a natural pace without clock-watching. If that means fewer postures, so be it. Allow at least four minutes for each posture you add to a sequence.

What poses to include Think about how you want to feel at the end of a sequence. If you're practising before bedtime, focus on Inversions, Resting Poses, and those performed from a reclining position. If you want to feel revved up for a night out or a meeting, add more Standing Poses.

Group your postures When building your own DIY sequence, this helps to keep the sequence smooth. If you jump from standing to sitting to inversions to standing to sitting, you will feel like a yo-yo, completely all over the place.

Think about counterbalance After practising yoga for a while, you will naturally start to sense which postures should come after each other, and how to 'counterbalance' movements with certain types of resting postures. If you twist one way, then of course you complete that posture by twisting the other way. This way of thinking informs yoga sequencing on a bigger scale, too: if you arch your back for Bridge Pose (see page 92), for instance, it

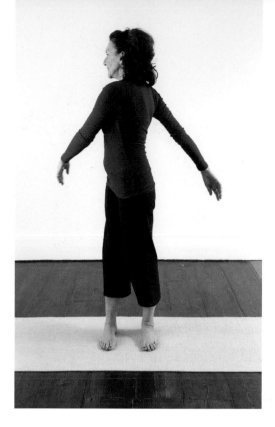

Start a yoga session by swinging your arms gently from side to side, T'ai Chi-style, to awaken the spine

can feel fantastic to lie on your back and hug your knees to your chest. Listen to what your body needs. Yoga will soon make that obvious, because it's all about getting rid of the mental clutter so that messages can get through, loud and clear.

Allow yourself to rest This is important in every sequence, whatever its purpose. Allow at least five minutes relaxation at the end of a 30-minute sequence (25 minutes of yoga, five of rest); take ten minutes during an hour's session. This is not cheating yourself; without relaxation, many of the benefits of yoga just don't accrue.

If you feel tired at any point during a practice session, give yourself a break and go into a resting pose like Child Pose (see page 118). Or lie on your back and hug your knees to your chest, rocking slightly from side to side. Remain there until you feel ready to continue. (Yoga is not a competition.) If you feel out of breath at any point, again take this as your cue to relax in a Resting pose for 6–12 breaths. In a class, too, there is no shame in dipping into a relaxing posture when you feel you need to. Listen to your body as well as to what your teacher is saying.

Sample home-practice session

Warming up: try this T'ai Chi-style warm up: stand in Mountain Pose (see page 60), then twist from the waist for 1–2 minutes, allowing your arms to slap loosely against your body. Then roll your shoulders and gently rotate your neck.

Standing Poses: these tend to be the most physical part of a programme.

Balancing Poses: to engage your brain and concentration as well as your muscles.

Core Strengthening Poses: to build strength and awareness.

Forward-bending Poses: these can be calming as well as provide a good stretch for the whole back of the body.

Backbending Poses: to open the chest and work on posture.

Sitting Poses and Twists: these categories are usually grouped together.

Inversions: the poses suggested in this book are safe for beginners.

Resting Poses: you could also include relaxation and breathing techniques (see page 152).

Herbal Eye Pillows

Eye pillows are among my favourite yoga 'props'; placed over the lids during deeply relaxing postures, they stop the eyelids from flickering which, in turn, helps to still the mind. They make wonderful gifts, too. Your herbal pillow should last about a year; renew it when the next lavender harvest is in. If for any reason you don't like the smell of lavender, make an unscented version by substituting sesame seeds for the dried lavender flowers.

2 rectangles (each 22cm x 13cm) of silky or
   natural fabric (cotton or linen)
150g flaxseed
50g dried lavender flowers
6 drops essential oil of lavender (optional)

Eye pillows stop the eyelids from flickering which, in turn, helps to still the mind

1 Pin the two rectangles of fabric together, 'right' sides facing. Stitch a 1cm seam around the two long sides and one end of the pillow, either by hand or using a sewing machine.

2 Turn the pillow case right-side out.

3 Put the flaxseed and the lavender flowers in a bowl, add the lavender essential oil (if using) drop by drop, stir to mix and, using a funnel, pour the mixture into the bag.

4 Stitching by hand, neatly sew the remaining side of the pillow closed.

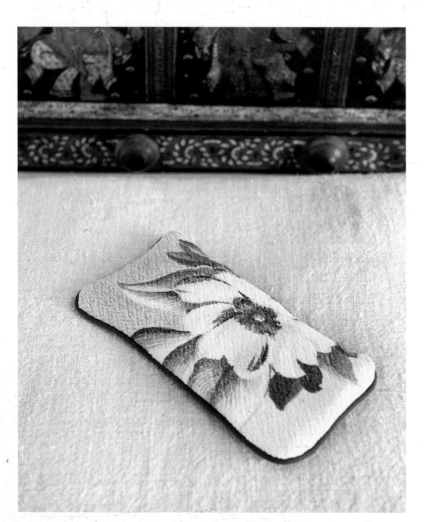

Allow yourself to rest. This is important in every sequence, whatever its purpose. Without relaxation, many of the benefits of yoga just don't accrue

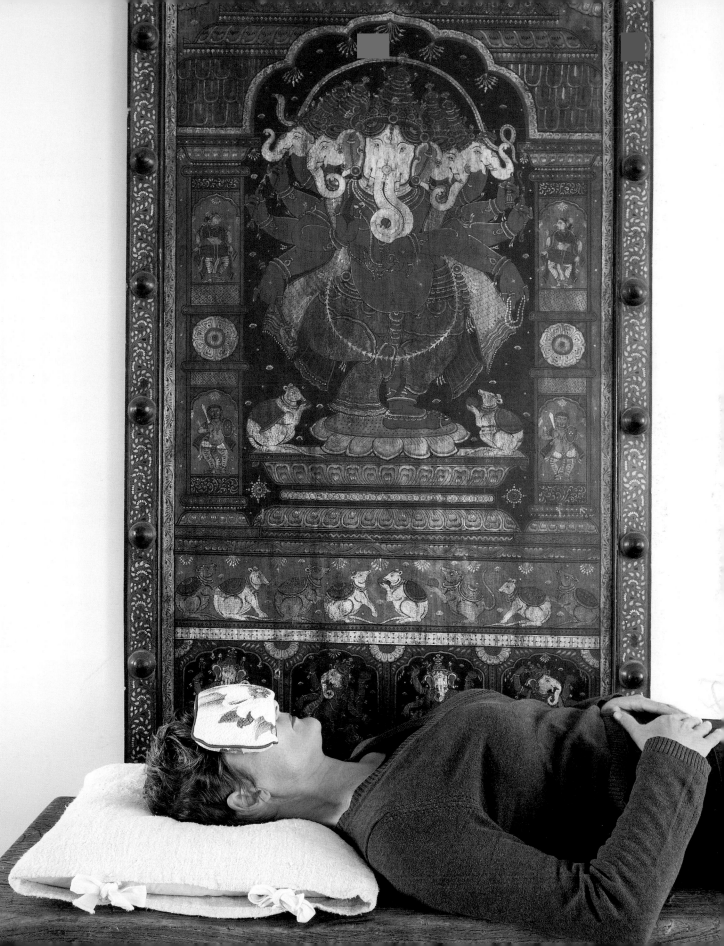

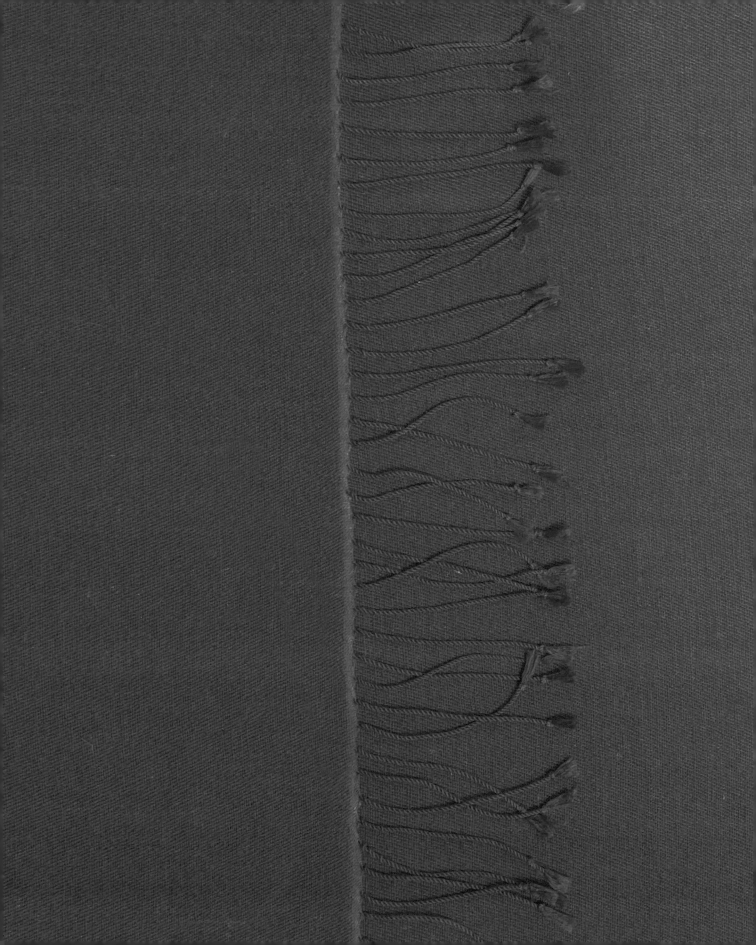

CHAPTER SIX

TOTAL RELAXATION

In the 21st century, 'more' is truly a four-letter word: our days are dominated by ever longer to-do lists, with more projects to finish, more meals to cook, more events to go to. Not to mention more, more, more electronic mail to deal with.... It is hardly surprising that so many of us feel crunched for time – and stressed. One of the greatest bonuses of a yoga practice is that it encourages us to stop the world and switch right off. In fact, if you get nothing else out of this book (and boy, I hope you do), then my wish is for you to introduce yoga's key relaxation pose (the slightly gloomily named Corpse Pose) into your too-much-to-do-in-too-little-time typical day.

It's safe to say that for many of us who enjoy yoga, the relaxation at the end of a session is almost the only time in a busy week that we get to lie down and do absolutely nothing. And it's not just allowed; it's encouraged. The danger is that before we know it, we've fallen properly asleep (and we've all done it), then wake ourselves snoring. But if you fall asleep during Corpse Pose – the concluding pose in most yoga sessions – then you're missing a fantastic opportunity to practise the art of letting go. There's even a Sanskrit name for this, pratyahara, which is defined as 'the conscious withdrawal of energy from the senses'.

Ironically, teachers will often tell you that Corpse Pose is actually considered one of the hardest poses for Western students of yoga to master. Just how hard can it be to lie there with your eyes closed? Once you've tried it, the answer's quite clear: it can be pretty tough, because we're so darned unused to it. We have become 'human doings', rather than human beings. Often paying the price with our health, since chronic stress can contribute to digestive problems, high blood pressure, heart trouble, insomnia and more. Not to mention wreaking havoc with our mental health.

Which makes relaxation – settling regularly into Corpse Pose – extremely valuable for our well-being. While we're apparently doing nothing, the body rapidly starts to heal itself. Blood pressure and heart rate drop, and the immune system is strengthened. (Yes, after just a few minutes.) Frazzled nerves are soothed, and furrowed 'thinking lines' on the forehead melt; muscular tension is relieved. As you sink into the mat (and into the floor, and the ground), your body starts to absorb all the good from your practice. I like to imagine it all 'sedimenting down' as I lie there, as if my practice is literally being absorbed into my muscles and bones.

Yet you often see people slink off their mats at the end of the active part of a class, skipping Corpse Pose with the excuse that they don't have the time. And, of course, it's people who think they have no time for relaxation who actually need it most.

So I'm about to make a bold proposal here: that even if you don't manage any other yoga postures during a day, you reward yourself every single day by setting aside 15 minutes for relaxation. Try it mid-afternoon, for example, as an alternative to drinking a coffee or a tea, and observe the impact it has on your feelings of

This is schmaltzy, but think of it as a gift to yourself – actually, not just to yourself, but to your family and those around you

well-being. This is schmaltzy, but think of it as a gift to yourself – actually, not just to yourself, but to your family and those around you. We're generally bad at taking care of ourselves, but I like the analogy with that important step in the oft-ignored in-flight safety instructions: before you put an oxygen mask on a child, put it on yourself. Translated to life on terra firma, this means: until you've looked after your own well-being, you can't look after others. So in order to gain all these benefits, learn how to get into Corpse Pose and drop into stillness by following these instructions.

RELAX – JUST DO IT

After a poor night's sleep, or when you really need to feel grounded, there is nothing like spending 15–20 minutes in Corpse Pose. As I've mentioned elsewhere, yoga has the spooky power to change the nature of time, in my experience: 15 minutes spent in relaxation is like begin given 30 minutes back, because you emerge better able to focus or think your way clearly through a challenge. Conversely, Corpse Pose can also be great for unwinding before bedtime. Don't practise in bed, though; place your mat next to the bed, so you don't have much of a journey to slip between the sheets when you're ready.

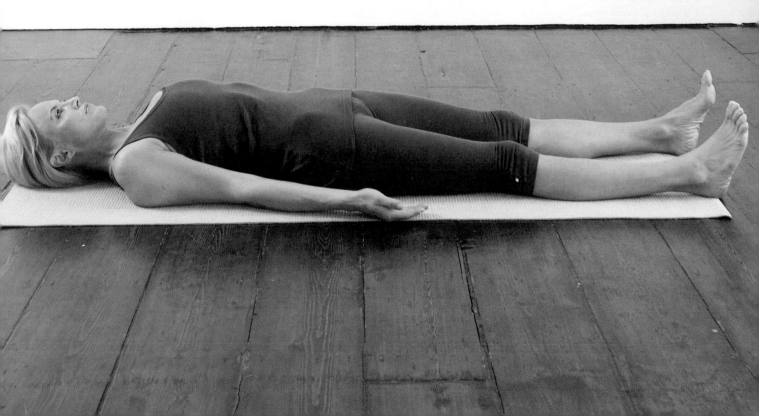

Corpse Pose (Savasana)
RESTING: BASIC

Because you are lying on your back to relax with your eyes closed, it is helpful to make a recording of yourself reading these instructions, or ask a friend to read it out. Be sure to leave pauses between each instruction. This relaxation encourages you to focus on your breath, one of the most powerful tools we have to calm the body. Who hasn't been told, in the midst of a frenzy, to take a deep breath? When you start to use your breath as a calming tool, the parasympathetic nervous system calms down and overrides any fight-or-flight responses. Don't expect to maintain a totally calm mind throughout your relaxation, though. We all find ourselves following trains of thought and filling out to-do lists. The mind can be like a disobedient puppy! Don't get agitated about this, just note it and return to your relaxation without judging yourself. However, I would be lying if I didn't say that some of my best ideas come to me in relaxation, to the point where I've almost been tempted to keep a small notebook by my mat!

TO START... make sure your mat is in a warm, quiet place. Except on a really hot day, it can help to close the window, to muffle distracting sounds. Have a blanket handy. It's extraordinary how swiftly the body cools, even after a vigorous class. You may feel warm as you lie down initially, but chilliness is not relaxing. You may even want to pull on a pair of socks at this stage. Have a timer ready (on your phone or an alarm clock) to ring at the end of the practice. If you find a bolster, eye pillow, folded blanket or towel useful, have them within easy reach. After the first few times you'll know exactly which props help you achieve total comfort.

Say to yourself in your head, 'My feet are relaxing. My feet are now deeply relaxed. My calves are relaxing. My calves are now deeply relaxed.' Move up your legs in this way, then focus attention on your arms, then your hips, chest, neck and head

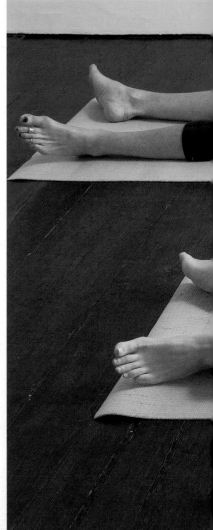

The body rapidly cools down during relaxation;
make sure you've got an extra layer on

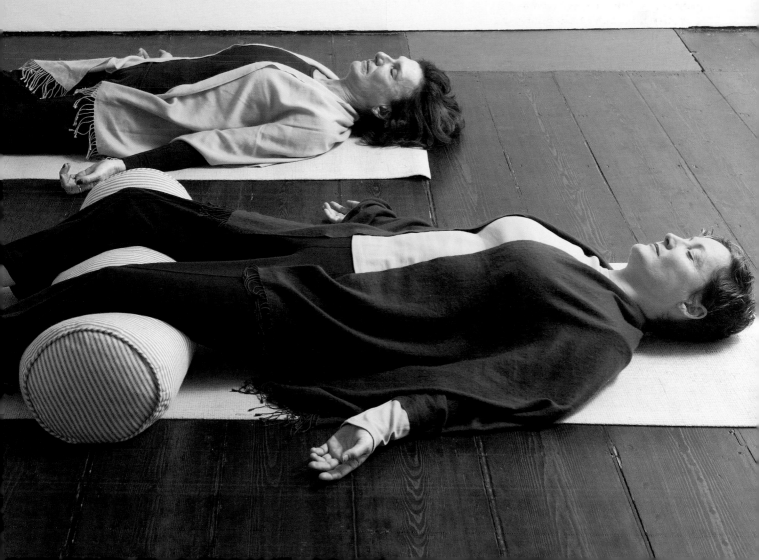

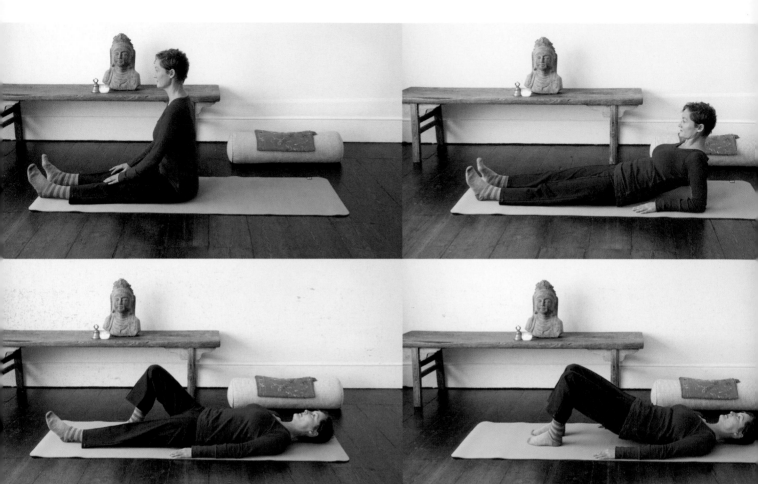

1 Sit up straight with your legs straight out in front of you and aligned.

2 Lean back on your elbows. Make sure once again that your upper and lower body are perfectly lined up. Then lower your upper body to the floor, one vertebra at a time.

3 Raise your hips, bend your legs and lengthen your spine. Rest your sacrum (the top of the pelvis) back on the floor evenly, and straighten one leg at a time, so they are hip-width apart. As you begin to relax, your legs will flop out slightly from the hip sockets.

4 If your lower back is uncomfortable, try placing a bolster under your knees. This is also better for knees that tend to hyperextend (a yoga teacher will tell you if this is your habit).

5 Roll your shoulder blades outwards slightly. You should now be lying with your hands about 15cm away from your hips, palms upwards and soft.

6 Check your alignment again. Lift your head, briefly, and make sure your chin, chest and navel are all lined up. As you lower your head back down to the floor, stretch the back of your neck slightly.

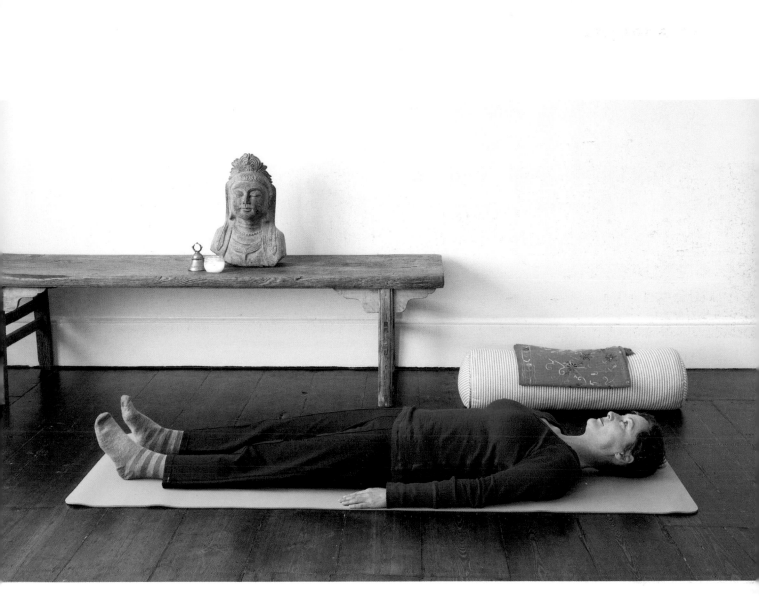

If your forehead is lower than your chin when you place your head gently back on the floor, try placing a slim folded blanket or towel under your head; your chin should drop below the level of your forehead. Cover yourself with a shawl or blanket if needed. This sounds like a lot of fidgeting, but it's worth getting right.

7 Start to release your arms, wrists, hands, legs and feet completely and deeply. Imagine you are 'earthing' yourself. For some people it helps to use a mantra that focuses, in turn, on different parts of the body. Say to yourself in your head, 'My feet are relaxing. My feet are now deeply relaxed. My calves are relaxing. My calves are now deeply relaxed.' Move up your legs in this way, then focus attention on your arms, then your hips, chest, neck and head. As you silently repeat the phrases, you can focus on those body parts, letting any tension ebb away. This doesn't work for everyone, but many people find it helps to still the 'monkey-mind', which is the real obstacle to stillness for most of us.

8 Soften your cheekbones, relax your jaw and your tongue. You may be amazed at how much tension you were carrying in your jaw.

9 Imagine your eyes settling in their sockets. If you have trouble relaxing your eyes, experiment by placing an eye pillow gently over your sockets. (There are instructions for making one on page 124.) The weight of the pillow can stop your eyes from flickering distractingly, and it bathes them in total darkness.

10 Keep your mouth closed and breathe through your nose. Despite the fact that the face is relaxed, an amazing beatific smile can often be seen on people in Corpse Pose, as if radiating like this is our default mode.

11 Allow your breath to rise and fall in your belly. Don't breathe shallowly through your chest; feel your breath way down in your belly. You'll probably be aware that the sound of your breath, as you do this, is rather like a gentle wave flowing and retreating on the shore. If it's helpful to hold that vision, go with it.

12 Most people find that they start to relax and 'drop down' into a quieter space after consciously following less than 20 breaths. At this point, you should start to feel increasingly quiet and peaceful.

13 When your mind starts to wander and chatter, as it will, filling with those to-do lists or ideas, still the voices by feeling your weight surrendering into the support of the earth beneath you. If you need to, repeat that body-part mantra, or have a go at observing your thoughts without reacting to them, almost as if they were clouds drifting by in the sky.

14 When you're ready, bring your awareness back to your body. Take some deeper breaths. Make a few small movements, wiggling your toes and fingers. You may want to stretch out completely, then flop down again.

15 Bend your knees and roll onto your side. Rest your head on your hands, then after a minute or two, use the strength of your arms to push you up to a comfortable sitting position. Keep your head relaxed, and look straight ahead.

16 Finish with a namaste (a traditional Indian greeting or salutation upon parting, literally meaning 'I bow to your form'): bring your palms together at heart level in prayer position, and bow your head. Take a moment or two to tap into how you feel. If you like, use this moment to send positive energy out into the world: to your loved ones, to colleagues or those in trouble somewhere in the world. Maybe it doesn't do a thing, maybe it does, but it certainly feels good.

17 Now get up carefully, and try to take some of the calmness you feel back into your everyday life.

Do... Be very kind to yourself, when starting out. Don't beat yourself up if you emerge after 5, 10, 15 minutes of relaxation without having mentally switched off. Simply resting your body has done it a massive favour. And there's always next time. ... Set a timer, preferably a quiet alert on your phone such as a pinging bell, to let you know when time's up. One major hindrance to dropping fully into relaxation at home is not knowing how long you've been lying there.

Don't... Worry if you don't switch off completely. In general, it gets easier to switch off as you practise, though at times of personal crisis or life overload, it can still be a huge challenge.

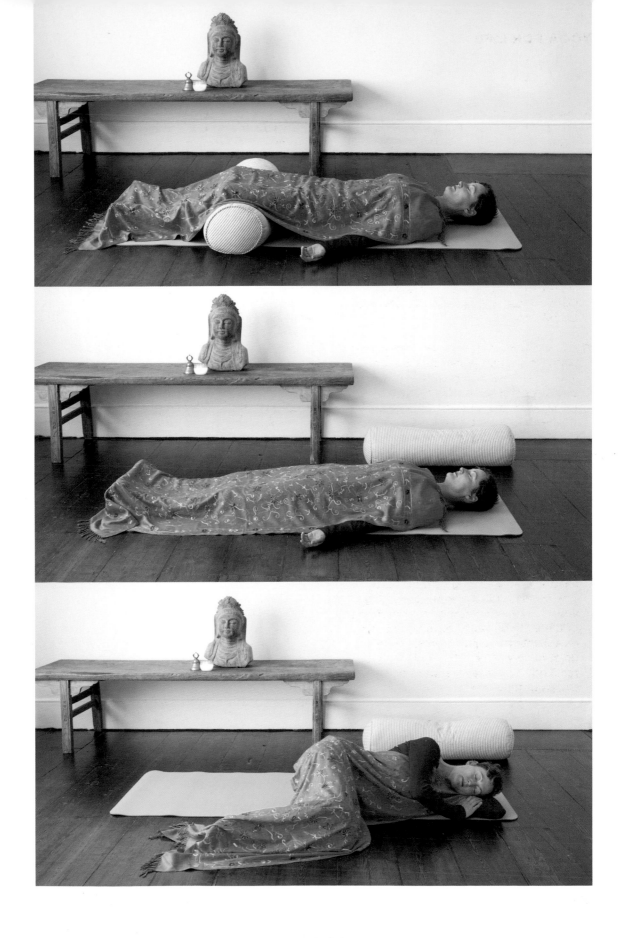

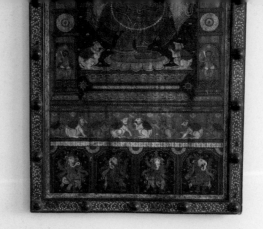

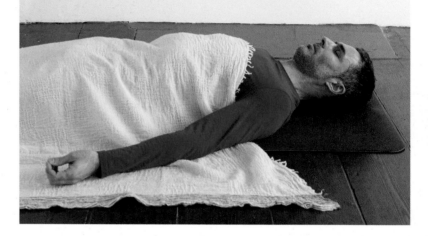

'When the breath
wanders the mind
is unsteady. But
when the breath is
calmed the mind will
be still and the yogi
achieves long life'

Hatha yoga proverb

The three stages of relaxation

There are actually three stages to Corpse Pose. The first is physical relaxation, which takes around 15 minutes. To begin with, in this stage, you're likely to feel that your mind is still racing, and be aware of thoughts and your physical body (itches, aches and pains). Gradually, though, your brain waves slow down and your blood pressure starts to drop.

During the second stage of relaxation, you'll no longer feel so conscious of what's happening in the outside world. Sounds and sensations no longer disturb you; it's as if they're happening further away. Thoughts stop whirling, or maybe you just find it easier not to get caught up in them.

Ultimately – and this is the true destination of relaxation – the mind lets go completely. At this point, it's believed that brain waves slow down to their lowest waking frequency. But it doesn't always happen. Some days you'll get stuck in stage one, though you should give yourself time to sink into the second stage every single day, if possible. The third stage is like being given the most fantastic present, but for all sorts of reasons it may not happen that often. Just appreciate it when it does.

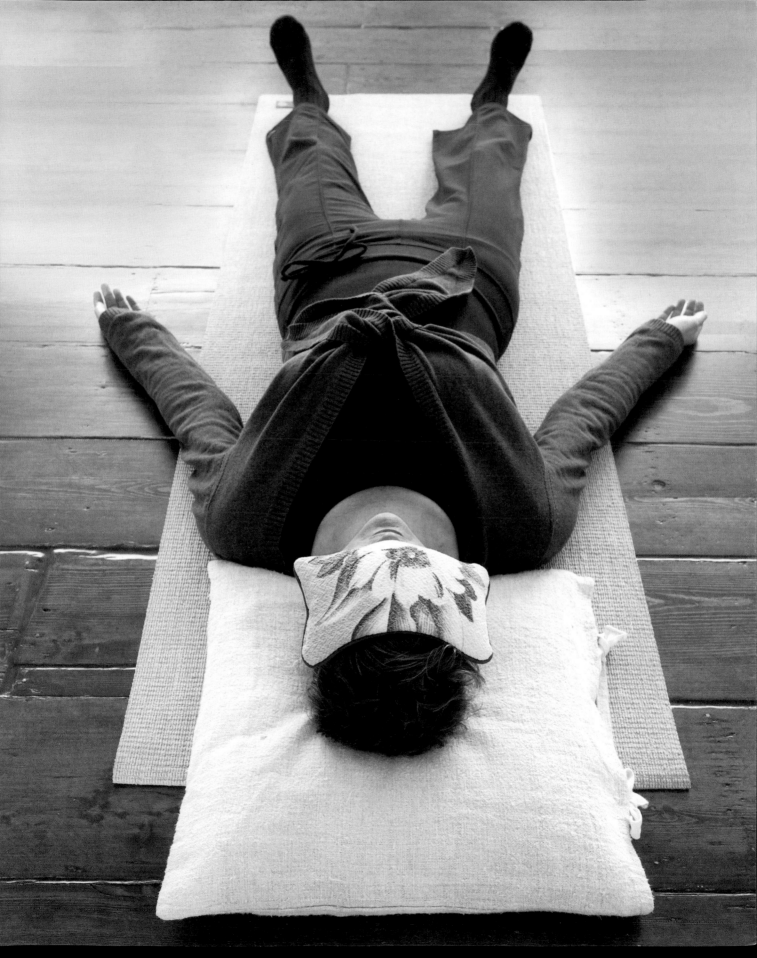

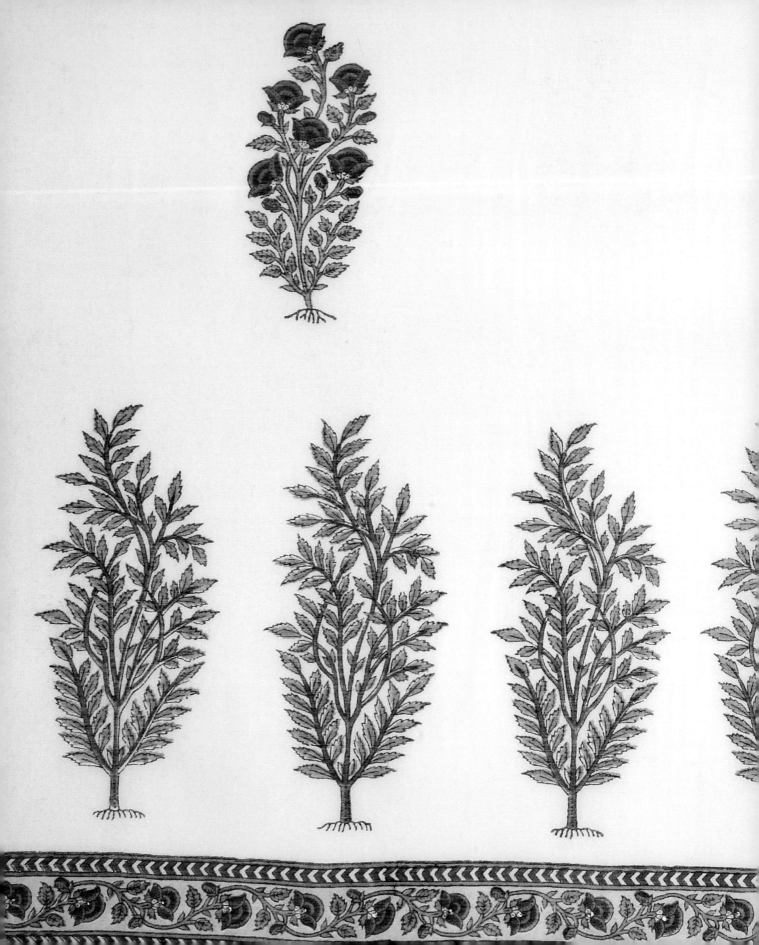

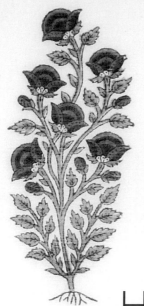

CHAPTER SEVEN

HOW TO FIND
INNER CALM

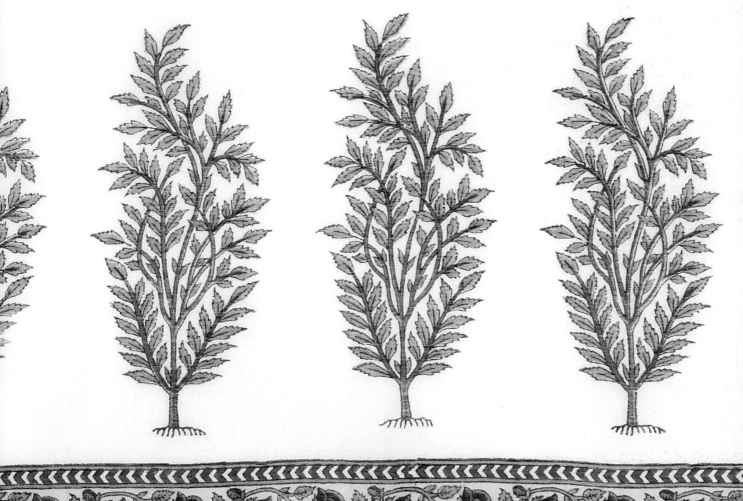

Originally, yoga was – above all – a spiritual practice. For many people, it primarily still is. Many others come to the mat wanting not just to stretch their bodies but to quieten the 'monkey mind' that is such a widespread side-effect of our too-much-to-do-in-too-little-time lifestyles.

Personally, I like the spiritual side of yoga. I find a lot that resonates with me. I have even developed something of a fondness for Indian deities: there's a Ganesh (the 'remover of obstacles' elephant god) on the top of my computer, plus a teeny Lakshmi (goddess of 'abundance'). But I've also found that rabbiting on about the spiritual side of yoga can be off-putting for many people (especially if they have a strong faith of their own). So – may the god/s forgive me! – I have mostly left out the spiritual side of yoga, in this book, to focus on the physical.

But then there's meditation. This is the closest many students will get to the 'spiritual' side of yoga, and it often opens up a new side to this ancient practice that you might want to explore further (there are plenty of book recommendations on page 221). For me, meditation helps me to find answers to some pretty big questions (along the 'meaning of life' lines, actually). I find that it also helps hugely with problem-solving. In general, only when I remove myself from the hurly-burly of day-to-day life do I get blinding realisations about what I should or shouldn't do in a particular situation. Meditation helps me to accept what life throws at me. And now that I've got the hang of it, meditation also promotes a sense of total calm.

That wasn't always the case. Trying to meditate used to make me feel furiously angry. And I'm not the only person I know who felt like that. In reality, meditation doesn't come easily to anyone. Even when you've had a brief, tantalising glimpse of how good it feels to tap into inner calm, clarity and connectedness, it can still be fiendishly hard to sit still and just 'be'.

If you have taken up yoga for its physical benefits, you might find that meditation makes you feel uncomfortable. It can feel like the 'woo-woo' side of yoga, and not everyone wants to buy into that, even though (according to the ancient sage Pantanjali), meditation – dhyana – is one of the eight essential 'limbs', or aspects, of yoga. But meditation absolutely totally doesn't have to be religious: nobody's asking you to become a Buddhist or a Zen monk, let alone swear a vow of chastity or poverty. You do not have to be a Beatle to meditate, or a movie star. Even if, famously, John, Paul, George and Ringo did head off to India to learn meditation from the Maharishi. And even if advocates include Goldie Hawn and Clint Eastwood...

THE BENEFITS OF MEDITATION

Over the years, a huge body of research has built up extolling the virtues of stilling the mind, which it is impossible to ignore. Meditation has also gained in respectability and credibility. In 2010, for instance, the Mental Health Foundation, the UK's leading mental health charity, declared that meditation should be prescribed routinely for depression (at the moment, only a handful of doctors do this). A study by researchers in Wales, Toronto and Cambridge found that in cases of recurring depression, meditation reduced the risk of relapse by more than 50 per cent.

Practised regularly, meditation is now also thought to keep at bay a wide range of complaints, including headaches, migraine, asthma, eczema, PMS, hypertension and even heart attacks. One London study of meditation and relaxation training for men and women at risk of coronaries found that, four years on, not only did members of the meditating group have lower blood-pressure readings, they also showed fewer symptoms of heart disease, less angina and a lower number of deaths from heart attack. (Can't argue with that.)

Meditation is also the most wonderfully natural and free antidote to the stress epidemic that's sweeping the world. It helps us deal with that stress by bringing about actual physiological changes that help our bodies, not just our minds. During meditation the heart rate slows, blood pressure normalises, and stress hormones (which wreak all sorts of damage in the body) are reduced. Sweating is reduced, too. Frankly, what's not to love?

WHERE TO START

Well, as I say, the act of meditation may be less-than-adorable, to start with. Just because meditation is simple doesn't mean it's easy. When I first tried to meditate, my mind was like an entire troupe of chimps reciting laundry lists, snatches of conversations, magazine-article ideas: it seemed that the very best way to start my mind racing was to sit cross-legged and try to meditate. The simple fact is that meditation is about effortlessness. What really transformed my experience was meeting a guru (yes, a real-life guru, albeit an American ex-hippie by the name of Ram Dass), who taught me two important tricks. First, that each time a thought came into my mind, I was to imagine it as a cloud and watch it drift away in my mind's eye.

Secondly, Ram Dass liked to use a small bell, which he'd ring at various points in the meditation to help us re-focus our thoughts. I realised that a bell resonates somewhere deep inside me: the vibrations help centre and focus me. That's entirely personal to me (although it might work for you, too), but what it made me realise is that for each of us there is usually a 'trigger' to help us go deeper into meditation. For you that might be a gong, perhaps, background chanting or the scent of a particularly grounding, earthy incense.

If you stick with meditation, you will almost certainly encounter what those of us who meditate regularly experience: a transformed mental landscape. You may not have to over-think or deliberate any more. When it comes to solving problems, the answers may come more easily. Old upsets may become more distant and less relevant, while the future (and all that we have to do) becomes less urgent. And when we do rise to meet those life-challenges, somehow, it's all that bit easier. Will that be your experience, too? If you stick with meditation, I'd put money on it. It will also bring down your stress levels dramatically.

So here are some suggested meditations, to get you started. There are several different techniques to 'try on', to see which works best for you. And if none of these work, there's a three-minute meditation exercise on Nintendo Wii-Fit, which is better than not meditating at all, to my mind! As Richard Rosen, author of *The Yoga of Breath*, explains, 'Meditation is like exercising a muscle. First, it's a chore. Eventually, it's a pleasure.'

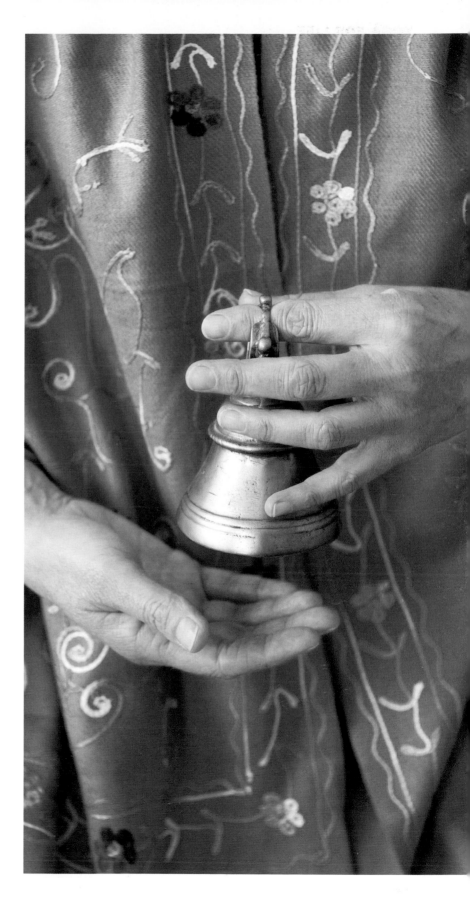

A basic meditation

Try to establish a regular time to practise this (and any form of) meditation. Early in the morning or last thing at night can be the easiest times to slip this into your routine, but try making meditation part of your yoga practice, if you have time. It can be wonderful to sit in meditation after your postures and before relaxation. Or after relaxation. See what works for you. Just don't attempt to meditate with a full tummy or when you're hungry. How often should you practise? As meditation teacher Hugh Poulton has observed, 'Just do it as long as you can afford – three minutes, 15 minutes, 30 minutes, twice a day. I see far more benefits in my students who meditate for five minutes a day, than those who do a long session once or twice a week. It's regularity that is the key.'

START BY... finding a quiet spot. If you have created a 'yoga space' for yourself, go there (see page 46). If not, find a room where you won't be disturbed. If you need to, hang a 'Do Not Disturb' sign on the door. Ticking clocks are hugely distracting (unless you decide that the sound itself is what you're going to focus on) so I recommend removing them. Then dim the lights or pull the blinds or curtains. It's easier to meditate when the lights are low.

1 Set a timer (or your phone) to alert you in five minutes. That's all the time you need to start with. It's extremely easy to lose track of time while meditating (or 'trying' to meditate), but if you know that there's a set time to stop, there's one less thing likely to distract you.

2 Make yourself comfortable. It may take a few attempts to find the ideal position. Sitting cross-legged can be comfortable at first, but if it feels like a bed of nails after a few minutes, extend your legs out straight in front of you. Try sitting against a wall, if your back gives you trouble when you sit upright. If you prefer, sit in a chair that supports your back, with your feet firmly on the ground (or on a stool if that brings your feet to a comfortable level). But don't get too hung up on the 'where': the best position for meditation is any one that helps you to stay focused. When you find that place, rest your hands in your lap, or in the traditional meditation mudra, or hand gesture: resting the backs of your hands on your knees with your thumbs and forefingers lightly touching. Or keep your hands in prayer position.

3 Notice your breath, allowing it to settle into a natural rhythm. Feel the air as it enters your nostrils, moving down to fill your lungs. Rest a moment and then let the air go gently, emptying your lungs. Try to breathe from your abdomen, not your chest, so that you feel your tummy swell as you inhale. Count to four as you inhale, rest for a beat or two, then exhale for a count of four.

4 To focus your mind and stop the flow of thoughts, try repeating a mantra: a favourite phrase, a word whose sound you love, even a line from a poem. Just repeat it over and over. A mantra doesn't need to have a meaning; it's the sound that helps you focus, tuning out the rest of the world. Try repeating your chosen mantra both silently and quietly out loud. (For a specific mantra meditation, see page 144.)

5 If the mantra doesn't work for you, try using images to still your mind. When you breathe in, visualise light filling your body from head to toe. And when you breathe out, imagine a darkness filling your body from toes to head. Alternatively, find an image from a magazine that you find incredibly restful; take a mental 'snapshot' of that image and focus your mind on it as you breathe in and out.

6 Keep coming back to awareness of your breath. Whenever a distracting thought breaks through into your meditation, simply acknowledge it and let it go. You might find yourself thinking about what you're going to do after your meditation. Or regretting something you've said to a colleague, or going over a scenario at work. As soon as you become aware of a thought, just say to yourself 'Thinking', and return your attention to the rise and fall of your breath. You'll probably find yourself doing this over and over during your meditation. It's normal to experience all states of mind – they arise and pass like the weather. Just don't get hung up on them.

7 Once the timer rings, bring your focus back to your body and the room around you. Gently move your fingers and toes, then have a stretch before getting up carefully. The next time you practise, slightly increase the length of time you sit for.

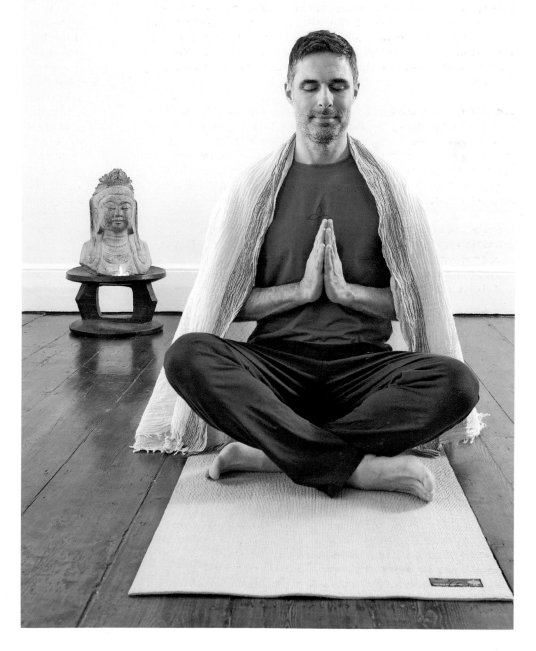

Do...

- Make yourself comfortable – this is absolutely the most important aspect of getting meditation to work for you.
- Pin any calming image you find useful for visualisation on a wall to 'refresh' your memory between meditation sessions.
- Make it regular. When it comes to 'successful' meditation, as with everything, the more time you put in the more likely it is that you will achieve what you are looking for.

Don't...

- Lie down to do your meditation, because sleep – while joyfully restful – is a thing apart from meditation. This is about slowing down, not shutting down, the mind.

'Begin to see yourself as a soul with a body, rather than a body with a soul'

Wayne Dyer

A mantra meditation

This meditation uses the power of sound and vibration to create stillness in the body. Traditionally, the words come from ancient spiritual languages, such as Sanskrit. Mantra-meditation teachers believe that the sacred meaning of the words helps to establish a connection to profound truths that have been spoken for thousands of years. Others believe that the vibrations the words have in the body produce the powerful effect...

This mantra meditation – and the sounds you repeat in the Walking Meditation on page 146 – are based on the Sanskrit syllables sat (which translates as 'truth') and nam (identity). This phrase is said to help us identify with a universal spiritual truth, and to encourage negative emotional states such as fear, anger and doubt to fall away.

START BY... finding a quiet spot. If you have created a 'yoga space' for yourself, go there (see page 46). If not, find a room where you won't be disturbed. Then dim the lights or pull the blinds or curtains.

1 Set a timer (or your phone) to alert you in 3–5 minutes, then make yourself comfortable by sitting with your legs crossed or extended, against a wall or in a chair. Rest your hands in your lap, or in the traditional meditation mudra, or hand gesture: resting the backs of your hands on your knees with your thumbs and forefingers lightly touching.

2 Take a long, deep inhalation through your nose. As you breathe out, say an extended 'soot' sound (that's actually how sat is pronounced), followed by a short 'nom' (that's strictly how you say nam). Together, it will sound like: 'soooooooot nom'.

3 Inhale slowly and evenly again. Repeat the mantra as you exhale, and continue with this rhythm.

4 Once the timer rings, hold your breath for a few seconds. Then exhale through your nose. Do this three times, then sit quietly for a few minutes and just feel the energy moving through your body. Open your eyes and carefully stand up. Carry that sense of calm and clarity with you throughout the rest of your day.

Do...

- Try taking a few drops of Australian Bush Flower Essences Meditation Essence (see page 220) before starting any meditation session, which really seems to work at preparing and calming the mind, and 'centring' you.

Don't...

- Limit yourself to ancient Indian languages. Use any words that inspire you and fill your heart with joy: 'Shalom', 'Amen', 'Peace', 'Life'. Try each one on for size, tuning in to how the vibrations you create saying the word make you feel physically.

'Meditation can take place when you are sitting in a bus, or walking in the woods full of lightness and shadows, or listening to the singing of the birds, or looking at the face of your wife or child'

J. Krishnamurti

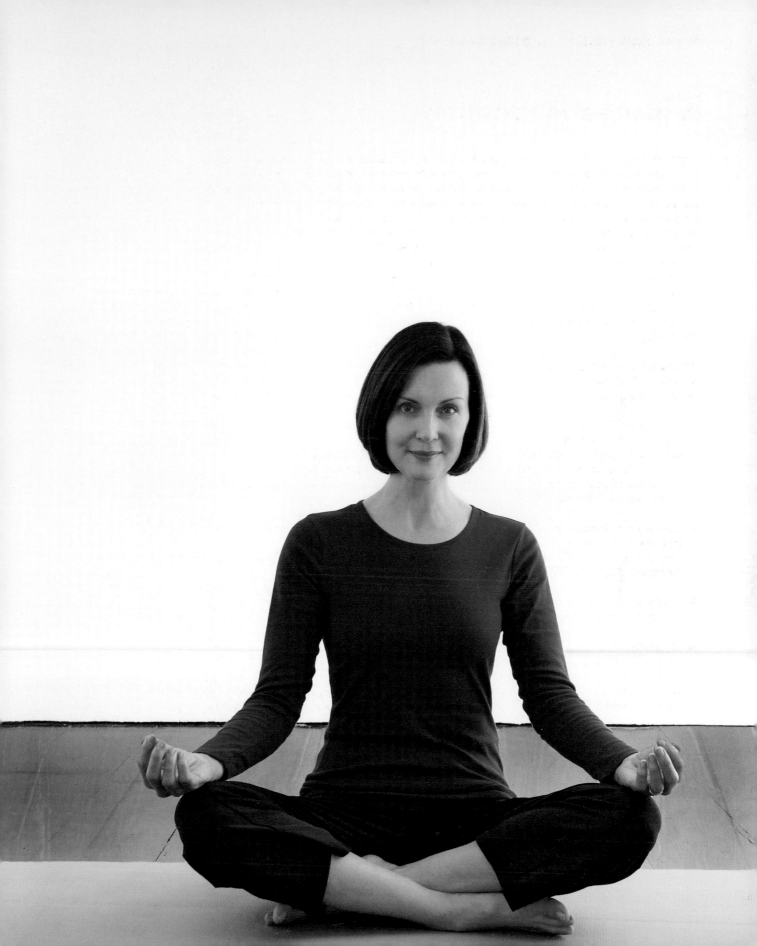

A walking meditation

If you find it hard to sit to meditate, experiment with a 'walking meditation'. For multi-taskers, it can seem like the perfect solution: a way to exercise and meditate at the same time, incorporating breathing (pranayama) and mantra techniques. Based on a technique used in Kundalini yoga (see page 34), this eight-minute walking meditation is energising. It's about 'being here now' and connects you with the earth. Try practising on a beach, in a wood, in a meadow or a city park. There's some really interesting research on this meditation technique at www.kundaliniresearchinstitute.org, where you can also find individuals who teach the method one-to-one.

START BY...walking at your natural pace.

1 Observe the sensations in your body: heat, cold, aches, pains, and so on. Even whether your clothes and shoes are rubbing or you're wearing enough layers. You may need to stop and make adjustments before you continue.

2 Tune into your breath. The optimum breath style for a walking meditation is even and regular, breathing through the nose and using the diaphragm.

3 Now try to match your breath to your stride. Inhale for four steps, then exhale for four steps.

4 When the matched breathing technique feels completely comfortable (and you may not want to move onto this stage on your first few walking meditations), make this adjustment: keeping your nasal passages and face relaxed, take four short, staccato puffs through your nostrils – one puff per step – to fill your lungs. (Don't breathe out between puffs.) After the first puff, your lungs should be roughly a quarter-full; after two puffs, half-full, and so on.

5 Exhale in the same way. Puff out roughly a quarter of the air in your lungs on the first step, and so on, until the fourth puff exhales the last vestiges of air from your lungs. This requires a little concentration. But that's the marvellous thing: because you're concentrating on your breath and matching the breath to your steps, it's almost impossible for the mind to wander. Continue this puffing in and out for about five minutes, then return to walking (and inhaling/exhaling) normally, for another three minutes.

'To transform the world, we must begin with ourselves'

J. Krishnamurti

6 Start the eight-minute sequence over again. But this time introduce a mantra: say the Sanskrit syllables 'soo ta na ma', with each step and each 'matching' breath. ('Soo ta na ma' literally translates as 'Birth, life, death, rebirth.' Big concepts for little words!) Repeat the mantra for five minutes, and again, return to walking (and inhaling/exhaling) normally, for another three minutes; you can continue silently saying the mantra, if you like, or just focus on the walking.

Do...

- Build up to the breathing technique if you tend to breathe from your chest or with an open mouth. As you get going with the walking, start by trying to breathe from your belly and through your nose.

Don't...

- Practise this meditation on busy streets, when you need to retain maximum alertness for crossing the road.
- Give up on the mantra. It's not that easy to co-ordinate, to begin with – but soon come, soon come, as the yogis say. According to Gurucharan Singh Khalsa in the book *Breathwalk* (see page 221), 'Practice for three days in a row and you'll feel the energising, focusing effects immediately. If you do it for 40 days you can really get intimate with the technique, and slip it into the cracks of your day to support you.'

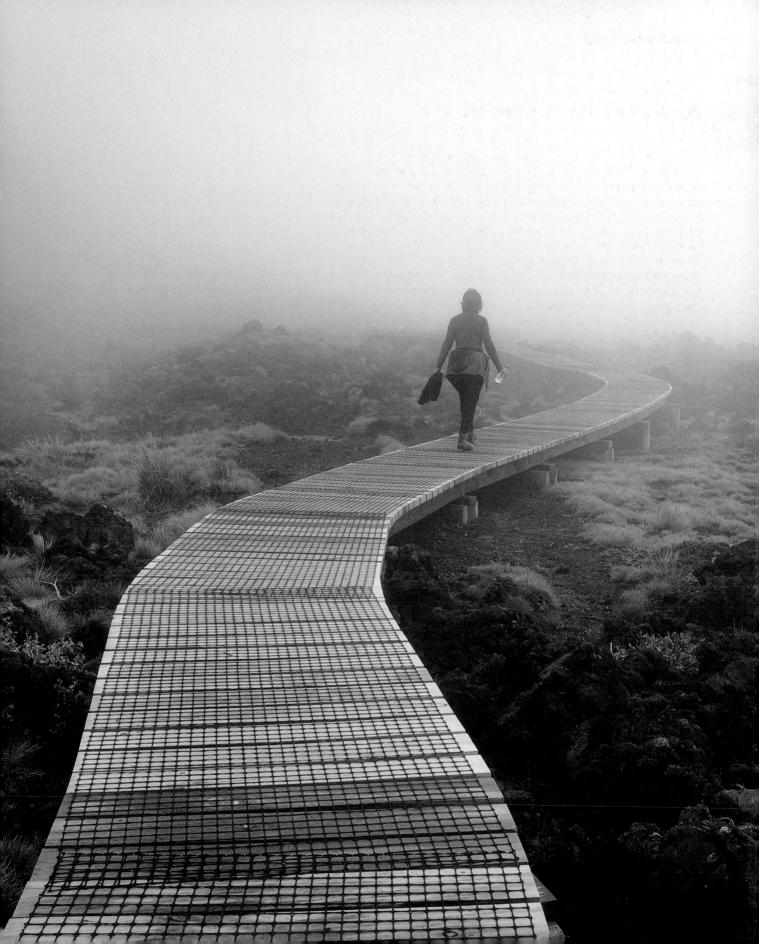

A healing meditation

This meditation focuses on chakras: the seven subtle energy centres thought to be situated along the length of the spine. Each chakra is associated with a different type of energy and is related to different states of being, and this meditation allows you to start exploring those more subtle, energetic aspects of a yoga practice. If this thought is a bit way out for you at the moment, stick with the Basic Meditation on page 142.

START BY... finding a quiet spot. If you have created a 'yoga space' for yourself, go there (see page 46). If not, find a room where you won't be disturbed. Then dim the lights or pull the blinds or curtains.

1 Make yourself comfortable by sitting with your legs crossed or extended, against a wall or in a chair (or on a bolster). Find what works for you. Rest your hands in your lap, or in the traditional meditation mudra, or hand gesture: resting the backs of your hands on your knees with your thumbs and forefingers lightly touching. Alternatively, for this meditation, you can lie on a blanket or yoga mat in Corpse Pose (see page 130).

2 When you're comfortable, try to imagine the stress melting away, and focus on your breathing, allowing it to become deeper and more regular. Be aware of the passage of air flowing into your body. Sense your heart beating, and visualise your body in its sitting or lying position.

3 Now it's time to imagine a rainbow-coloured iridescent energy, or prana, being taken into your body along with your breath.

4 Take your focus to the base of your spine. This is the position of the 'base' (or muladhara) chakra. Envisage a whirlpool of iridescent energy swirling there, and, at the same time, try to imagine the earth's grounding energy being drawn up into you.

5 Next, focus on a point in the small of your back, about 7cm above the first chakra. This is called the swadisthana chakra, and when we're subjected to stress of any kind, it's felt here. This chakra also relates to the unconscious mind, which is why we almost 'feel' things in this part of the body as we tap into our instincts. Imagine the iridescent energy revitalising this particular area for a minute or so.

6 Now focus your attention on a point about 3cm below your navel (the manipura chakra), and allow your breath and the iridescent prana energy to energise this area.

7 Move your focus up, to the area in front of the heart. Visualise the energy flowing both in and out of the heart chakra here; some teachers believe this is where spirit, soul and body meet.

8 Next, take your focus and the iridescent energy to a point in the front of your neck, halfway between your shoulder blades and your chin. This chakra – vishuddha – is linked with communication. Those-in-the-know maintain that this chakra has a blue energy, and they advise wearing blue around the throat when public speaking, to enhance the power of your words. Hold your focus here for a minute or so.

9 Move upwards to focus on a point just above your eyes, behind your forehead – the ajna or famous 'third eye' chakra, responsible for deep insight and intuition. At this point, let yourself relax totally. Aim to spend four or five minutes imagining that golden iridescent energy revitalising this chakra, bringing you into balance.

10 Last, but not least, it's the turn of the crown, or sahasrara chakra: concentrate on a point 1–2cm above the top of your head. Visualise the whole of your energetic body (not your physical body, but the aura around you), shining with a bright white light.

11 Try to conjure up an image of the universe itself, and draw that powerful energy down towards you from the heavens, until it merges with your own bright white 'halo'. Imagine that white light flowing down through the crown chakra, energising your whole body with its healing energy. Hold this thought for a few minutes.

12 Visualise all the energy from all the chakras drawing into your physical body, then gradually re-enter the world. Wiggle your fingers and toes and stretch. Lastly, open your eyes and slowly unfold from your seated position, giving yourself a good stretch.

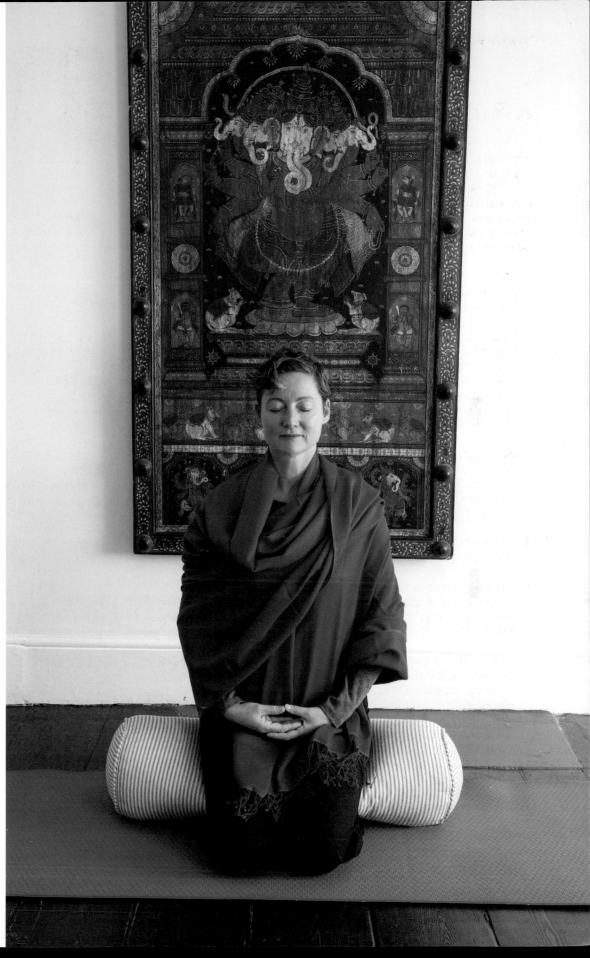

Do...

- Be gentle on yourself after practising this meditation. Drink a glass of still water and take it easy for a while.

Don't...

- Be concerned if you find this technique too other-worldly. Go back to whichever of the other techniques worked for you – whichever helped to de-furrow that brow will be the best.

A study found in cases of recurring depression, meditation reduced the risk of relapse by more than 50 per cent

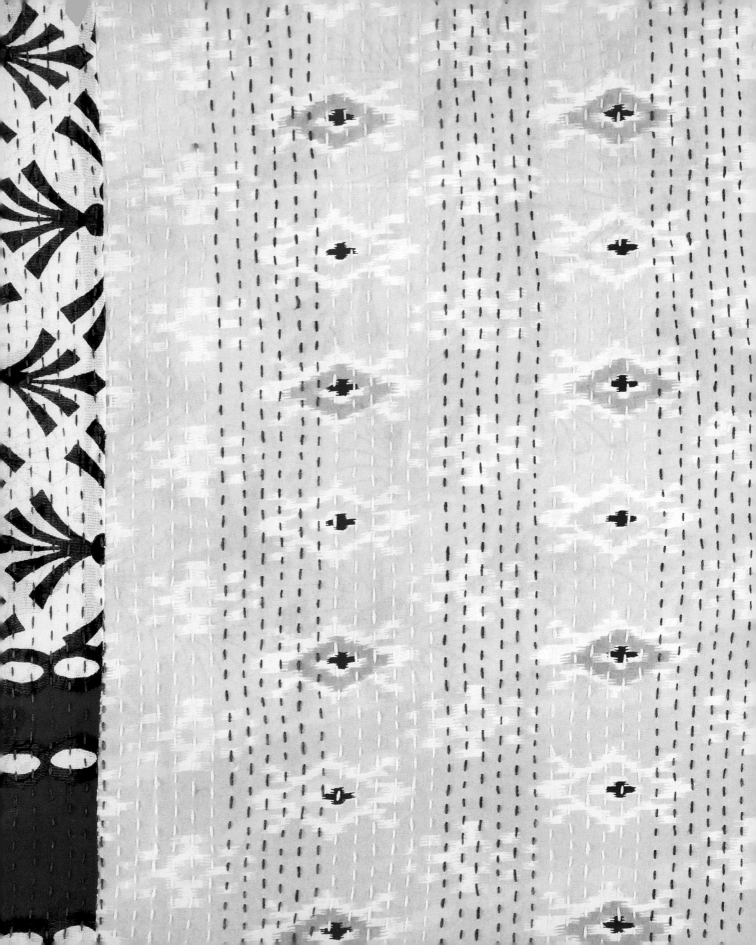

CHAPTER EIGHT

THE MAGIC OF BREATH

We talk about something being 'as natural as breathing' – and yet when we start to do yoga and focus on the breath, sometimes it doesn't feel natural at all. In fact, we're generally so unconscious of breathing that when we have to think about it and control it, we become quite stressed.

Breathing, though, is so darned miraculous – our body takes in air and that keeps us alive. Wow! That is surely worthy of awareness and attention. Being 'on the mat' is the perfect opportunity to find out more, especially since the correct breathing, matched with movements, can actually make some postures easier. What's more, there is a specific yoga breathing technique – pranayama – worth exploring in its own right, as a tool for relaxation and clearing the mind.

Different styles of yoga, of course, recommend different styles of breathing. Astanga teachers, for instance, teach a technique called Ujjayi (say it 'yoo-jie') breathing, which means 'victorious' breath: a strong, almost rasping breath from the back of the throat (see page 156). If you start Iyengar yoga, meanwhile, there may not be much focus on breath at all at the beginning, until you've got the hang of the postures. In class, follow your teacher's instructions. And don't be judgmental. There's no 'best' way to breathe. But there are some basics – here they are:

Don't hold your breath A no-brainer? Not a bit. It is really, really common to find that while concentrating hard on a posture, you've been holding your breath unconsciously. So keep focusing back on your breathing, 'checking in' with it throughout your practice.

Think: steady, rhythmic, smooth Calm, even breathing quickly instills a sense of calm – and this 'yogic' breathing is something you can access at any stressful time. Keep your inhalations and exhalations the same length. Mentally count them, if you're unsure: use a count of four as you breathe in, a count of four as you breathe out. It works like magic to drop you into relaxation: in bed, on the mat, on the bus, even.

Breathe through your nose, not your mouth The passages in the nose warm, purify and moisten the breath en route to the lungs, making it healthier always to breathe only through your nose. Occasionally in yoga, breathing through the mouth will be suggested though, for instance, in 'lion breath', when you roar like a lion, which is impossible through your nose!

If in doubt, reach for a tissue At home, always keep tissues handy near your mat – and you may like to tuck a couple into your yoga pants for class. Quite a few forward bends and inversions can make your nose run, and it's good to clear the passages before starting a class. Always blow your nose before pranayama (see below), to avoid feeling self-conscious about air 'whistling' through your nose!

As a rule of thumb, exhale when you exert yourself For instance, when coming into Shoulderstand (see page 116) or Warrior Pose (see page 66), do so on an out-breath – it's almost as if it helps to 'power' you into the pose.

Return to your regular breathing if it all gets too much There's a lot to take on board in any yoga practice – making sure you're aligned, getting your limbs in the right place, keeping your balance – and on top of everything, you're meant to breathe properly. If you feel overwhelmed and out of sync, just simplify things and return to your normal 'off-the-mat' breathing pattern; it's better than stressing out about whether you're getting it 'right'. The well-known Iyengar yoga teacher in the US, John Schumacher (a pioneer, who has taught yoga for almost 40 years), likes to say to his students with a wry smile, 'Breathe in on the inhale. Breathe out on the exhale.' Hah!

'Fear less, hope more; eat less, chew more; whine less, breathe more; talk less, say more; hate less, love more – and all good things are yours'
Swedish proverb

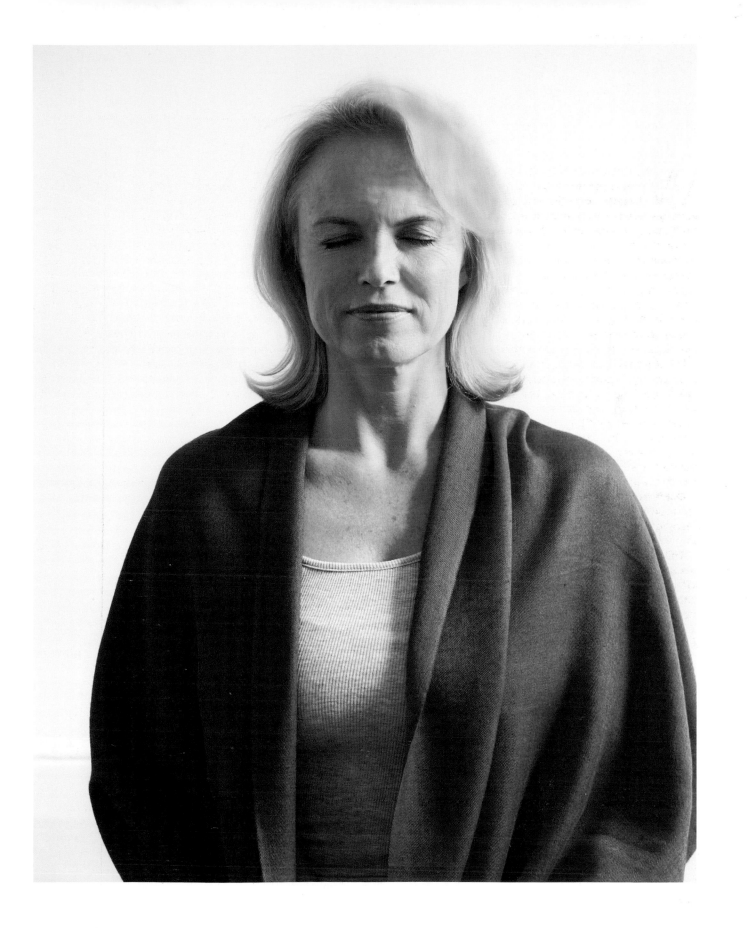

Breath of life

The Sanskrit term pranayama translates as 'control of prana' – and prana is basically our life-force, or energy. Pranayama isn't just your normal yogic breathing; it's a separate 'arm' of yoga, intended to clear and cleanse the body and the mind. It makes an especially fantastic preparation for meditation, helping to centre and focus the mind. And, you may hate it.

I've never been asthmatic, but the closest I have come to that panicked, can't-breathe feeling was when I first started practising pranayama in a class. In fact, it was enough to make me avoid that class again. And another class, when the teacher introduced pranayama. But I do understand that it's very 'unyogic' to dislike part of a yoga class as much as that. I had also realised, by that point, that one of the great benefits of yoga was to make us more flexible – not just physically, but mentally – and that I wasn't really entering into the 'spirit' of yoga if I just avoided the breathing element of yoga.

So, I stuck with it. And guess what? I really love pranayama now, most especially what it does to calm my 'monkey mind'. My effort (and it was an effort) paid off. I do know many other students who haven't got on with pranayama, so if you fall into that category, my advice is: stick with it, and you'll get it in the end. You may even actively start to enjoy it. And if you love it from the word go? Lucky you! Here are some basic pranayama exercises, to get you started:

Alternate-nostril Breathing (Nadi Shodhana Pranayama) Sometimes translated as 'sweet breath', Nadi Shodhana is thought to 'cleanse the channels' in the body, allowing energy to circulate more freely. It is a brilliant resource when you're stressed, helping to promote clear thinking and still the mind. Ten rounds is all it takes, I promise. It also makes the perfect final step before relaxation or meditation, and can help during your practice when you're feeling a bit off-kilter or are finding it hard to balance.

START BY... sitting comfortably cross-legged on the floor, against a wall or on a chair; alternatively, lie back supported by a firm bolster.

1 Hold up your right hand, then curl your index and middle fingers towards your palm. Take your palm towards your face, then place your thumb above your right nostril, and your ring and little fingers above your left nostril.

2 Close your left nostril by pressing gently against it with the tips of your ring and little finger. Inhale through your right nostril – make this a slow, steady, full breath.

3 Close your right nostril by pressing gently against it with the tip of your thumb, then open your left nostril by slightly lifting your ring and little finger; exhale fully – again keeping the breath slow and steady.

4 Now inhale through the left nostril, close it by pressing down with your fingers, and exhale through your right nostril. That's one round of 'sweet breath'.

Short guide

• Inhale through right nostril
• Exhale through left nostril
• Inhale through the left nostril
• Exhale through the right nostril.

Variation with a pause: Once you have mastered the basic technique above, try breathing in for a count of four, hold your breath for a count of four, then breathe out (through the opposite nostril) for a count of four. Follow the 'short guide' instructions, but just add in a pause after inhaling each time.

Do...
• Count slow 'beats', four in and four out. Or do what one teacher taught me: start with one beat in, one beat out (on both sides). Then count two beats in, two beats out; three beats in, three beats out, and so on, until you have worked up to one l-o-n-g ten-beat breath.

Don't...
• Overfill your lungs; the in-breath should feel natural.

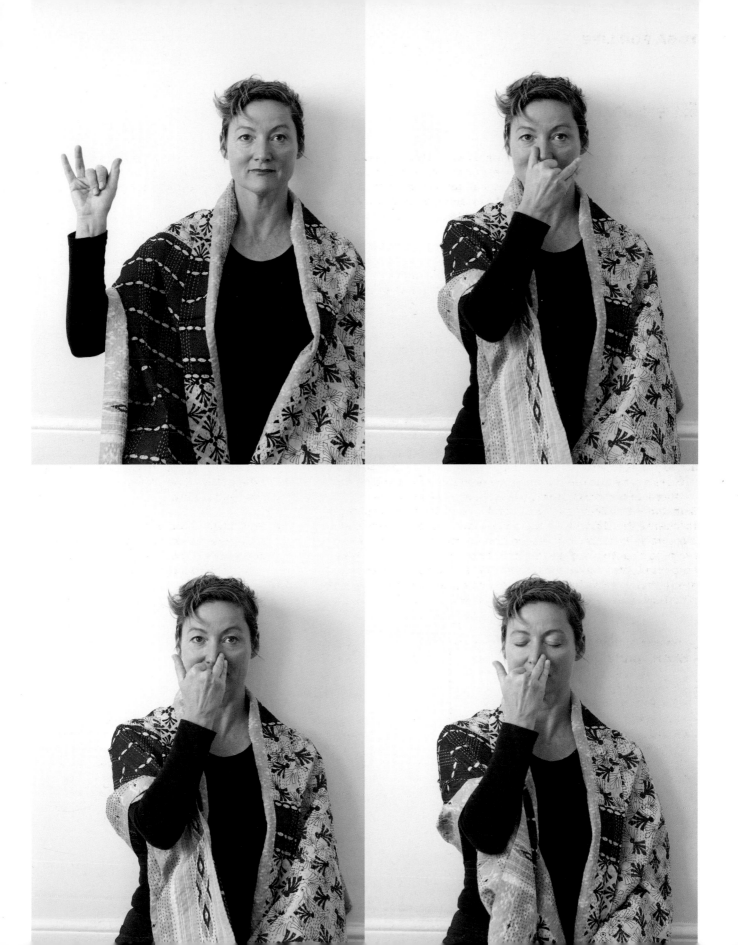

Ocean Breath (Ujjayi Pranayama)

Ujjayi breathing (say it 'yoo-jie'), also known as the 'sounding' or 'ocean-sounding breath' is, slightly more heretically, called Darth Vader breath, which is the best clue I can think of as to how it should sound when you do it right. It is good for focusing the mind: if you have a project to complete and you're finding it hard to rein in your thoughts, do some 'ocean breathing'. It increases mindfulness, so is good whenever your thoughts feel scattered. And it's also brilliant for building internal heat: on a cold day, Ujjayi breath is wonderfully warming.

START BY... finding a comfortable seated position cross-legged on the floor, against a wall or in a chair. Alternatively lie on your back – it can feel good to place a bolster under your knees.
.

1 Take a few long, deep, slow breaths in and out through your nostrils.

2 Slightly contract the back of your throat to make a hissing sound as you breathe steadily in and out. If someone came close, he or she would be able to hear your breathing.

3 Lengthen your inhalations and exhalations as much as you comfortably can, while still feeling relaxed and comfortable. While you're doing this, listen to your breathing; the sound alone can be as calming as one of those 'ocean wave' relaxation tapes.

Do...
• Try this during standing poses (once you feel comfortable with the technique) if you need to find focus.

Don't...
• Make a snoring sound; the sound is sort of en route to a snore, but not quite; it shouldn't be that forced.

'When you inhale, you are taking the stength from God. When you exhale, it represents the service you are giving to the world'

BKS Iyengar

Checking your technique

To be sure you're getting the breath 'right', hold your hand to your mouth and breathe out as if you were trying to fog up a mirror or a windowpane. To get the 'fog', you have to constrict the back of your throat. Now close your mouth and do the same thing, but breathing through your nose. That's Ujjayi breathing.

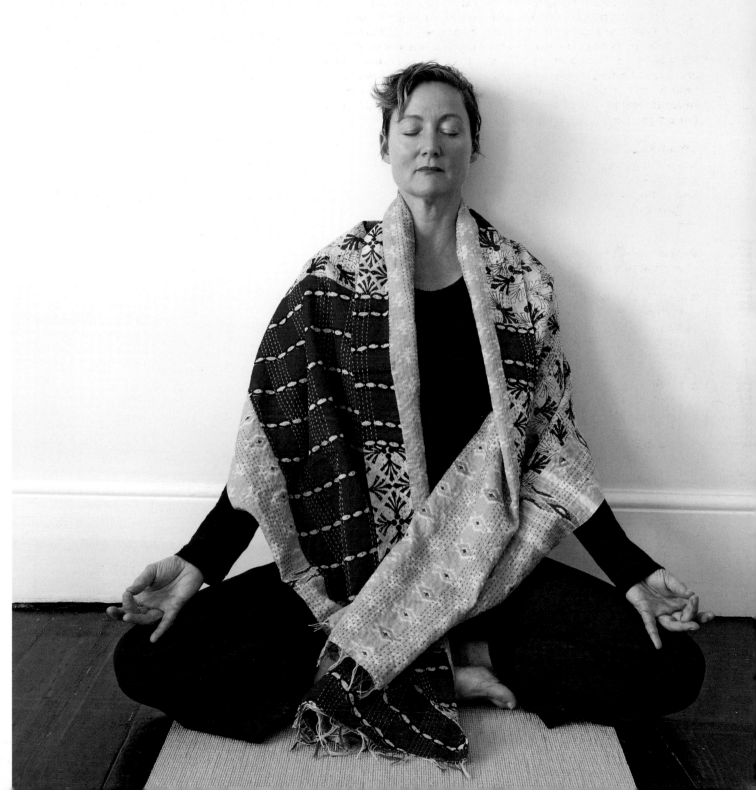

'Smile, breathe and go slowly'

Thich Nhat Hanh

CHAPTER NINE

YOGA FOR
THE BEST SLEEP
OF YOUR LIFE

'Sleep,' it's been said, is 'the sex of the millennium'. None of us, in other words, is getting enough. As a result, as many as one in twenty people in the UK turn to prescription pills, and we also try homeopathic remedies, herbs such as valerian, a couple of glasses of red wine.... And yet yoga, as many (including me) have discovered, is a far healthier prescription for getting a really good night's rest.

Happily, there is a simple yoga sequence that should ease you into restful sleep. Which is great, especially if you've been suffering from chronic insomnia. But the sleep challenge many of us share, at a certain age, is that we drift off fairly easily, but wake in the wee small hours, and start tossing and turning, unable to get back to sleep again. For women going through perimenopause and menopause, hot flushes can cause sweaty night-waking to fling off the covers. So here's what to do when thoughts are whirring at 3am and, in the dark, the world seems a scary place.

Pose-wise, inversions are said to particularly good for sleep issues. But if you have only just discovered the joys of yoga at mid-life, I don't believe that 'advanced' inversions like Shoulderstand or Headstand are to be recommended. I've just heard too many anecdotal accounts from no-longer-spring-chickeny acquaintances about how these two poses, in particular, have led to injuries. Better safe than sorry, is my mid-life yoga philosophy. Besides, Legs-up-the-wall Pose (see page 114) is easy and qualifies as an 'inversion', making the many benefits of Shoulderstand available in a pose that's accessible to all.

All the following poses, though, are excellent to build into a pre-bedtime sequence: they're calming, soothing and should bring down your pulse and blood pressure. In brackets you'll find the page numbers of the poses themselves, but there's some additional, sleep-related advice here about how to use props such as blocks and blankets to make the poses even more relaxing. Ideally, you should take a Yin yoga (see page 35) approach to these poses at the end of a day, moving slowly and thoughtfully between them and – when it comes to the lying/seated postures – stay in each for five minutes or so. That may feel beyond you when you start your yoga practice, but as the yoga gurus say, 'Soon come, soon come...'. Ideally, set your mat up near your bed and do these in your pjs.

I would recommend choosing three or four of these poses – why not your favourites? – to create a personalised sequence. Add to the sequence once it has become familiar. This will be most effective when it becomes a repeated ritual, since it then starts to trigger a relaxation response in the brain. If the sequence isn't working for you, mix it up a bit with some new postures, but give each sequence a week or two to become effective, letting the habit sediment down into your psyche.

Happily, there is a simple yoga sequence that should ease you into restful sleep. Which is great, especially if you've been suffering from chronic insomnia. These poses are excellent to build into a pre-bedtime sequence: they're calming, soothing and should bring down your pulse and blood pressure

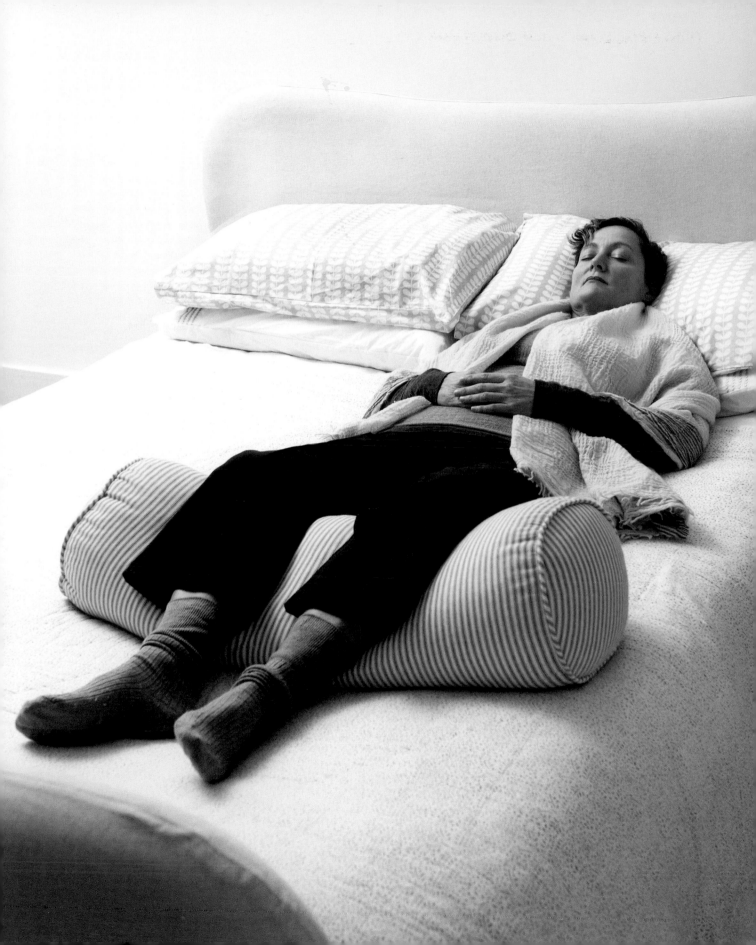

Poses to choose from

Standing Forward Bend (see page 80) Do this for a minute or so, but come up slowly so as not to feel dizzy.

Wide-legged Forward Bend (see page 84). This standing pose is actually one to turn to whenever you're feeling stressed or overwhelmed; it's very grounding.

Downward-facing Dog Pose (see page 64) Hold for as long as is comfortable. If you like, sink back into Child Pose (see page 118), rest for a minute or so, then repeat. And so on, for as long as you like.

Seated Forward Bend (see page 82) Place a firm bolster in front of you, between your legs, in line with your body, before you bend forwards. You need to sink completely into this posture to make it relaxing; if the hamstrings in the backs of your legs are so tight that relaxing forward is difficult, even with a bolster, just pile on some folded blankets or towels, until they're the right height to support you. There's an additional tip here, too: when you rest down into your pile of props, the skin on your forehead will probably squidge up one way or another; try to make sure it squidges downwards, towards your eyes, rather than upwards, towards your hairline. This helps to stimulate the relaxation response and also calm your nervous system.

Cobbler Pose (see page 88) Practise this one lying on your back – or try reclining back onto a firm bolster – with the soles of your feet together and drawn in towards your groin. Support your knees with blocks or folded blankets so you can let go of any 'holding' in the thighs. In this form, the pose is known as Reclining Bound Angle Pose.

Supported Reclining Twist (see page 108) Prepare for this pose by ensuring that the pile of blankets you relax into is high enough to support you without strain, so you can truly feel yourself sinking into the pose.

Legs-up-the-wall Pose (see page 114) This is one of the best poses when you can't get to sleep, especially if your insomnia is hormone-related.

Corpse Pose (see page 130) You can do this after you get into bed and perform what's called a 'body scan' while you lie in the pose: simply tense and then relax each part of the body in turn. Or mentally 'talk' yourself through a total body relaxation, starting with your feet and legs and working upwards. Just say to yourself, 'I am relaxing my left foot. My left foot is relaxed. I am relaxing my right foot. My right foot is relaxed…' and so on. This technique is especially effective for anyone who experiences 'mental chatter' the minute they close their eyes, since focusing on the body scan occupies the brain while slowing it down.

Supported Relaxation Pose (see page 120) Remain in this pose for 15–30 minutes at the end of your pre-sleep yoga ritual.

Return to slumber

To help yourself back to sleep in the middle of the night, try Legs-up-the-wall Pose and/or Corpse Pose. Corpse is easy to do in bed, and the 'body scan' technique can be very effective for helping you to get back to sleep (and done without disturbing anyone you share a bed with). If you are worried about waking your partner when you swing your legs up the wall, keep an area of wallspace in the bedroom clear so that you can slip out of bed and rest with your legs elevated for ten minutes. Keep a blanket handy, if the bedroom's chilly at night. This takes a little 'prep' before bedtime, but is so worth it. In my experience, it beats hands-down the traditional advice to turn on the light and read a book or do the ironing, because once that light's entered my brain, I'm wide awake. If you know the geography of your bedroom and can get into Legs-up-the-wall Pose in the dark (the usual health-and-safety warning about trip hazards applies), you may find this works better for you, too.

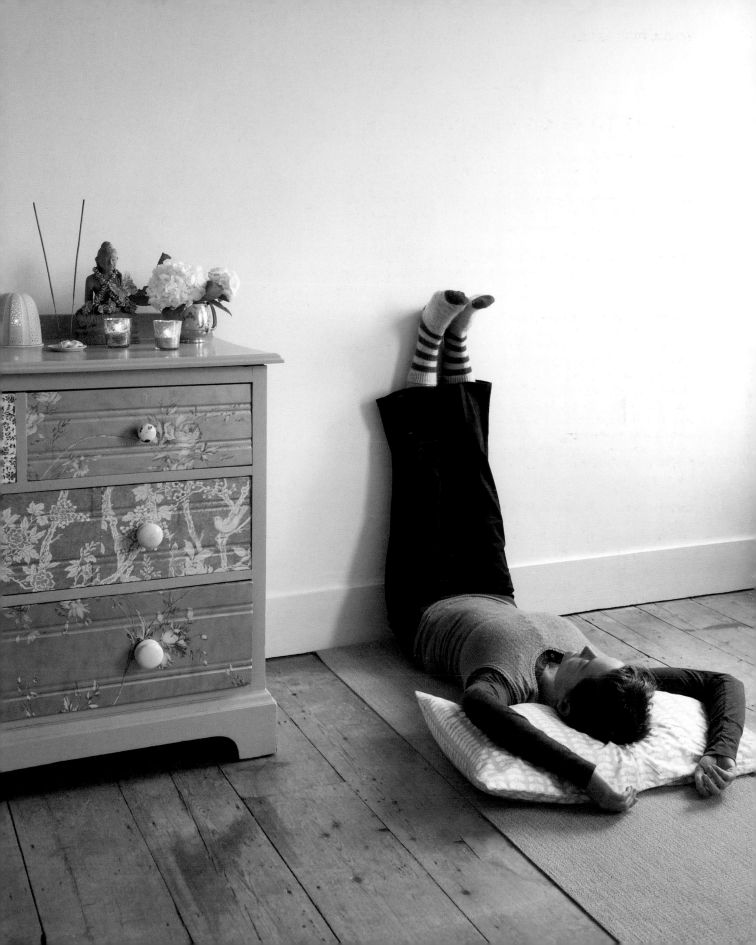

Other sleep-inducing strategies

Wind down before you put your head down To give bedtime yoga a chance to work, create a wind-down period before you hit the sack. You can't check e-mails till 10pm and expect to drift off when your head hits the pillow. Turn off the TV, computer and radio well in advance of bedtime, but especially iPads and smartphones. Research has shown that the light from these devices, which hits the pineal gland from relatively close-up, interferes with circadian rhythms and upsets your natural sleep cycle.

Look for a Yoga Nidra class Also sometimes known as 'Yogic sleep', or 'Sleep with awareness', this class sets out to induce full-body relaxation and a deep, meditative state of consciousness. You're not really asleep, but frankly, it's as restful as if you have been. If you can't find a class, encourage your favourite teacher to study Yoga Nidra and start offering it. Most yoga teachers are up for extra training; it's a discipline that encourages exploration and development. There are recommendations for Yoga Nidra CDs/downloads on page 220.

Breathe yourself to sleep Breathing is a really powerful tool for stilling mind and body. At the start of your pre-bedtime sequence of poses – or any practice when you've rushed to the mat – begin with some long, unhurried breathing, as per the following technique. You will find that just five or ten breaths help you to 'drop down' into a quieter space. It's downright miraculous.

START BY... swallowing, and consciously releasing the tension in your throat and belly. (You'll suddenly be aware of this.)

1 Close your eyes and begin to inhale evenly through your nostrils. Focus completely on the inhalation, and make it slow and long.

2 As your breath expands your lungs, let your chest lift and your ribcage expand. Feel your shoulders naturally widen. There shouldn't be any strain.

3 At the end of the inhalation wait a beat, and then exhale evenly through your nose. The 'in' and 'out' breaths should ideally be the same length; you can count to 'pace' them evenly.

4 Notice any changes in your body after you have completed one long breath. When you're ready, start again. Build up to at least ten long breaths maintaining focused concentration.

'We live in a chronically exhausted, overstimulated world. Yoga Nidra is a systematic method of complete relaxation, holistically addressing our physiological, neurological and subconscious needs.
Yoga Nidra uniquely unwinds the nervous system, which is the foundation of the body's wellbeing'

Rod Stryker

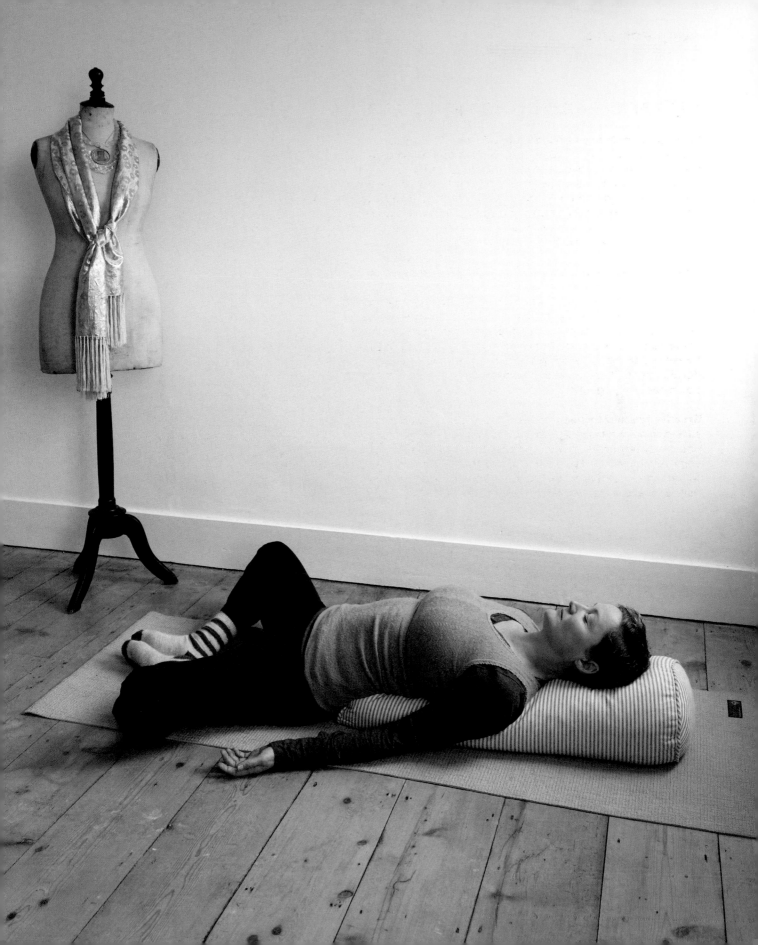

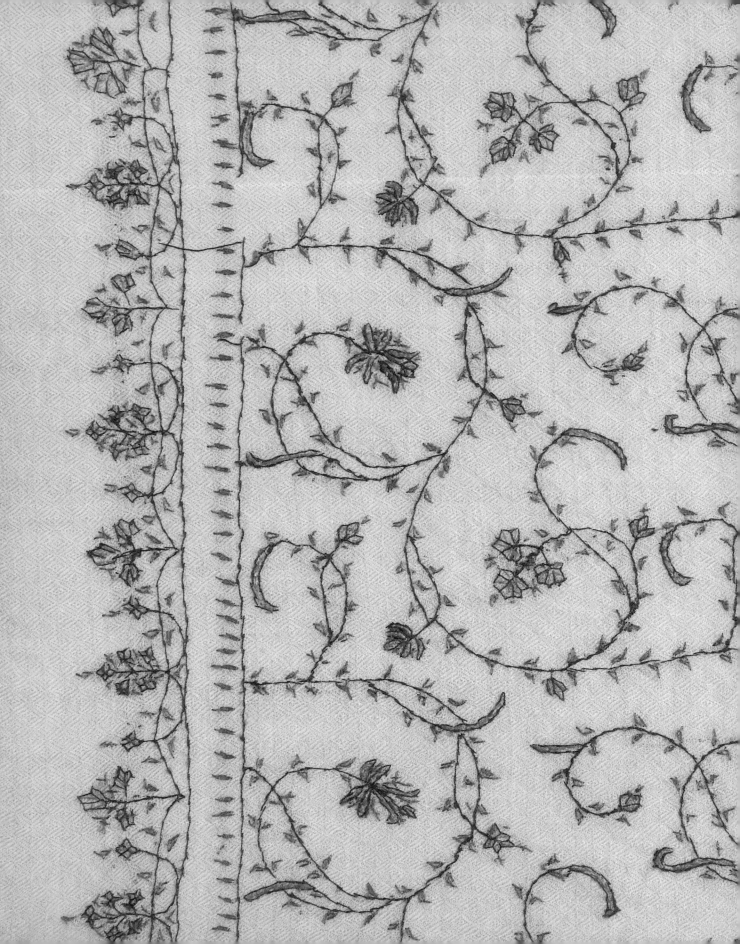

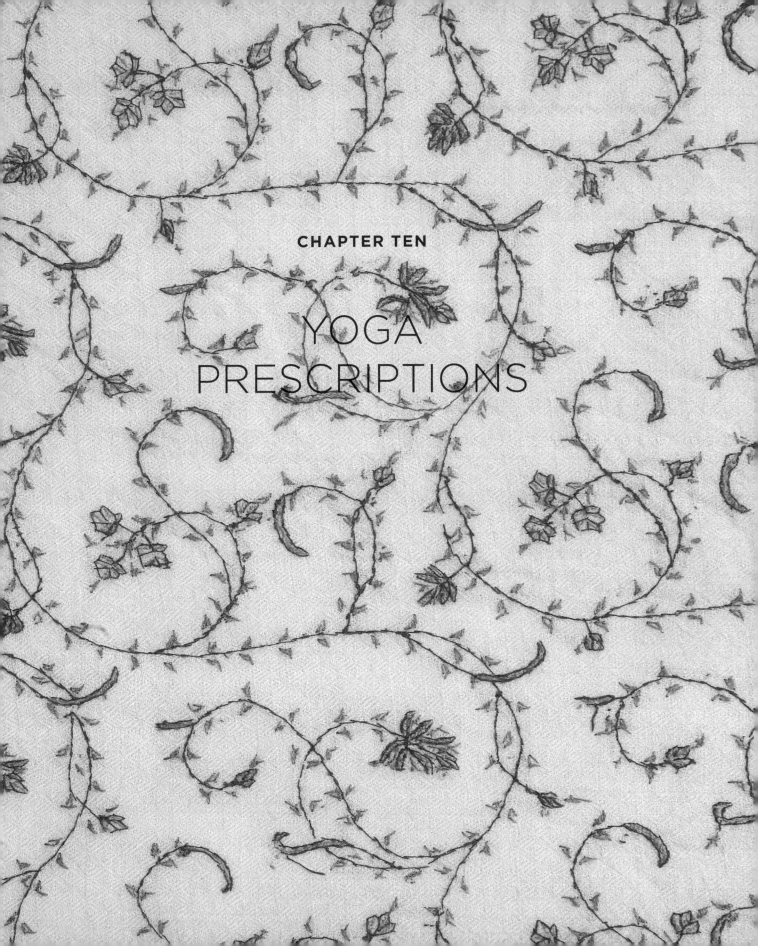

CHAPTER TEN

YOGA PRESCRIPTIONS

Yoga is much more than a way of exercising or quieting our thoughts in a crazy-busy world. It has also successfully been used to help various challenges that our minds and bodies face as we age. So on these pages you'll find some specific sets of postures that many, many people have found invaluable for different body issues. Of course they're not a substitute for seeing a doctor or a qualified health professional, but they are a way of helping to take charge of your own health – and you may find them very beneficial.

BEST POSTURES FOR MENOPAUSE

Hot flushes, sleepless nights, mood swings – these are among the many 'joys' of menopause for many women. Yoga can be a fantastic resource at this stage of life, because of its effect in balancing the endocrine (hormonal) system. The result of a regular yoga practice for many women is reduced symptoms. Of course, this varies according to the individual, but it's got to be worth a shot – particularly if, like me, you don't want to go down the HRT route.

If you're going through menopause, be sure to include the following poses as part of your practice. Many of them are 'inversions', which might seem counter-intuitive when the biggest nightmare, for many of us, is feeling 'hot and bothered' and inversions position the body completely or half-way upside-down. You might think that would make you even hotter and even more bothered – but anecdotally from countless women, the opposite seems true.

If you have high blood pressure, start with the very gentlest inversions, such as Seated Forward Bend (see page 82) and Legs-up-the-wall Pose (see page 114), which initially you should hold for just a few minutes. If you have any qualms, you may even want to discuss your yoga practice with your doctor, before practising inversions. And whether you have high or low blood pressure, always come out of inversions extra slowly and carefully on an inhalation. You need to avoid quick changes of pressure in the head, which can happen when you move from lying to sitting, sitting to standing, or coming out of an upside-down pose.

- **Downward-facing Dog Pose** (see page 64)
- **Legs-up-the-wall Pose** (see page 114)
- **Supported Shoulderstand** (and eventually, with a teacher, Shoulderstand) (see page 116)
- **Standing Forward Bend** (see page 80)
- **Big Toe Pose** (see page 86)
- **Seated Forward Bend** (see page 82)
- **Handstand** (I've not included Handstand in this book since you need to learn it under the guidance of an experienced teacher, and only after you have been practising yoga for some time.)

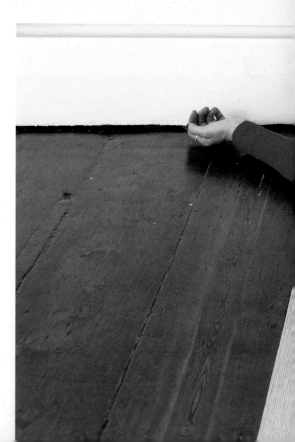

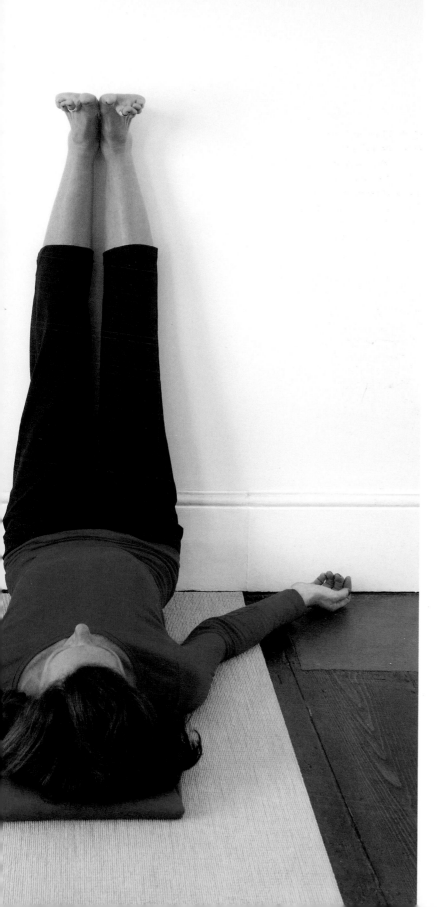

BEST POSTURES FOR STRENGTHENING BONES

The following postures, in particular, have been found helpful for building bones. If you're already showing signs of osteoporosis or osteopenia, however, be sure to explain this when you're with a new teacher. Iyengar yoga (see page 32) can be particularly helpful, because of its focus on alignment, posture and safety. You can't just 'throw' yourself into any old class: some postures are actually risky for osteoporosis sufferers. Forward bends, for example, can increase the risk of fracture, and twists put the spine in a vulnerable position. That's why it's always so important to talk to the teacher before a first class – ideally, in advance, so that you can gauge for yourself if the teacher understands the contraindications for osteoporosis. If you're ever nervous about doing something during class, speak up and get feedback from the teacher. And if in doubt, sit it out.

- **Tree Pose** (see page 70)
- **Chair Twist** (see page 102)
- **Bridge Pose** (see page 92)
- **Warrior I** (see page 66)
- **Cobra Pose** (see page 94)
- **Downward- and Upward-facing Dog Poses** (see pages 64 and 98)

QUICK FIXES

Yoga can also be a great short-term help for certain conditions. Use it to:

FIX A HEADACHE

Anecdotally, I have a couple of friends with a long history of migraines who've taken up yoga, and whose crippling headaches have disappeared. But headaches have many triggers: visual strain (from staring at a computer or failing to update a spectacles prescription), high blood pressure, or, it's now believed, just not breathing properly. There seems to be a link between 'upper chest' breathing and headaches, for some people. Regular yoga can change the way you breathe, re-educating you to use the diaphragm well, rather than relying on the chest wall and neck muscles. Yoga also opens tight areas in the chest or abdomen that may inhibit breathing, while correcting postural mistakes, such as the habit of jutting your chin forward and misaligning your head and neck when sitting in front of a computer screen. Better breathing can definitely prevent stress headaches, but can also lessen the severity of those that have already begun. If you've been parked in front of your computer and a headache's swooped painfully in, before you reach for a painkiller, try this:

MODIFIED FORWARD BEND

1 Stand behind the back of a high-backed chair and place both hands on the back.

2 Take a couple of steps away from the chair back and hinge forward from the hips so that your upper body is horizontal to the floor. Keep your knees slightly soft (don't lock them) and lengthen your spine. Adjust your foot position and start again, if you're too close to the chair.

3 Keeping your upper arms aligned with your ears, lengthen along the outside of your arms and your ribcage.

4 Keep your throat, tongue and eyes relaxed. Breathe deeply and slowly, holding the position for 10 breaths in and out. Return to the upright starting position, keep your eyes closed and imagine everything 'settling', like sand in an egg timer. Repeat, if you like.

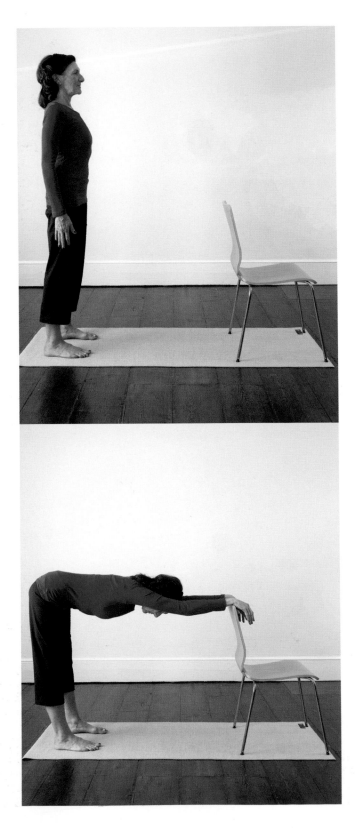

POSE FOR THE BLUES

A German study showed that emotionally distressed women became less depressed after they took two 90-minute yoga classes a week for three months. Dr. Andrew Weil, the respected naturopathic doctor, suggests, 'If you experience fatigue or mild depression, try Wide-Legged Forward Bend. It has many benefits, including for lack of energy and poor mood.' For full instructions, see page 84.

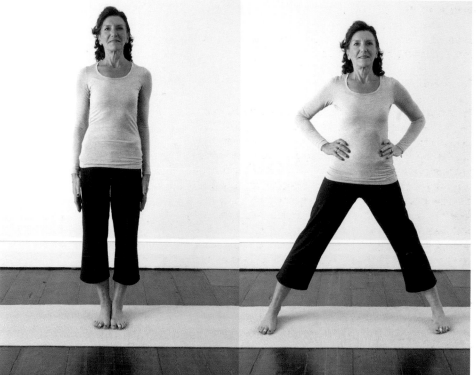

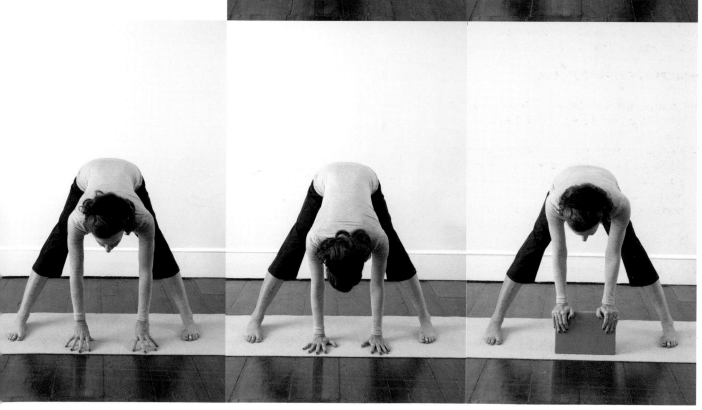

BETTER THAN A LAXATIVE?

In the chapter on pages 174–95, you can discover the art of eating well for yoga, with recipes for nurturing foods and calming teas, and a section on 'mindful eating' (many experts now believe this promotes weight loss more effectively than dieting). But because so many of us eat on the go, wolf down unhealthy snacks or skip meals, digestive problems like constipation, acid reflux, heartburn, gas and irritable bowel are all on the rise, particularly as we age, when digestion may just not be as efficient as it once was. Certain postures alleviate many of these problems. Twists, for instance, encourage 'peristalsis' – the involuntary relaxation and contraction of the muscles that move food along the digestive system. Twists also massage hard-working organs used in the digestive process, the liver, gallbladder, spleen and pancreas, while lessening gas and constipation. So instead of a laxative or a bowl of bran, try this:

Twists are extremely good for massaging the hard-working organs used in the digestive process – the liver, gallbladder, spleen and pancreas

SEATED SPINAL TWIST

1 Sit on your mat with your legs extended straight in front of you and your spine tall – in Staff Pose (see page 112). Fold a blanket and sit on the edge of it to tilt your hips forwards a little, if you find your lower back rounds in this position and you're hunching.

2 Cross your left leg over your right, placing your left foot flat on the mat close to your right knee. Bend your left leg to bring the foot as close as is comfortable to your right hip. If folding the leg over the other is uncomfortable, just bend the right leg and bring your left foot alongside the right inner thigh.

3 Place your left hand on the mat next to your left hip, and your right hand next to your right hip. Lift the crown of your head to lengthen your spine, while sinking down through your hips. (Keep your weight evenly distributed between both hips, rather than tilting to one side).

4 Exhale as you rotate your upper body to the right, reaching your right arm behind you and placing your fingertips on the mat.

5 Wrap your left hand around the outside of your left knee, and take hold of your thigh – or wherever it reaches comfortably. Don't strain.

6 Stay in the pose for up to 60 seconds, then slowly release your limbs and and twist to the left, so that both sides experience the benefits of the twist.

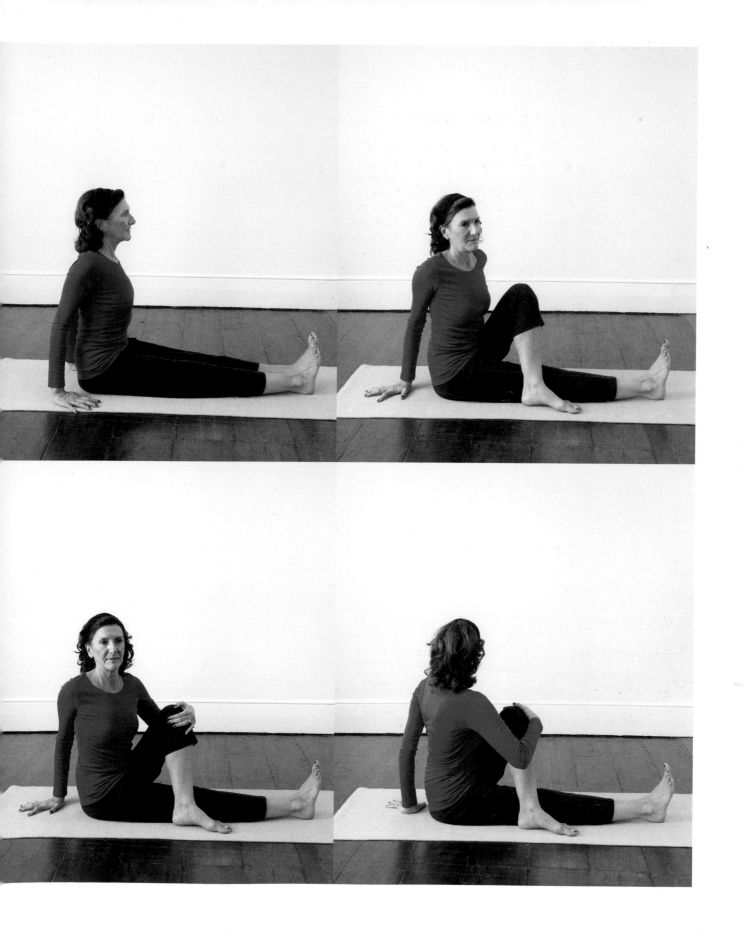

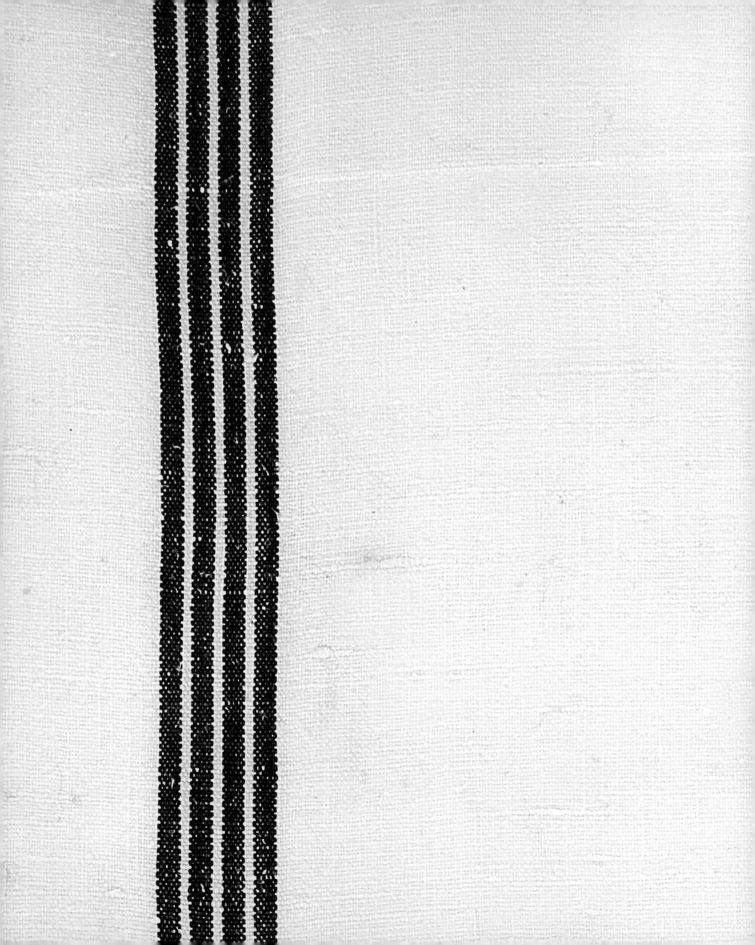

CHAPTER ELEVEN

THE YOGA OF FOOD

For almost everyone I know who's taken up yoga, the benefits have been many, varied and unexpected. And one area that can really undergo a shift is an awareness of what we eat and drink, and how it affects the body and mind, energy levels and mood swings. The knock-on effects of last night's large glass of red wine, for instance, may show up tangibly in extra wobbliness during a balancing posture. On the other hand, you might become aware that a raw-food salad you ate for lunch has left you feeling clear-headed and zingy, seemingly able to hold a tricky posture more easily.

Often, yoga works at a deep level, improving our relationship with our bodies – and uncomplicating a long-term relationship with food. As we start to observe the link between what we do, what we eat and how we feel – which can be disconnected when we're just hurtling from A to B with no sense of stillness – it can be easier to overcome even long-standing food habits and eating patterns, such as grabbing sugary, fizzy drinks to replenish energy, or hitting the biscuit barrel because we're feeling in need of TLC. As you gain a sense of harmony and balance (and truly, there isn't a soul I know who does yoga that this doesn't happen to), you may well find that your emotional relationship to food changes – because you're being sustained and energised by yoga. You start to eat to live, rather than live to eat.

What frequently happens, I've observed, is that people start to recognise what food their body actually needs, and when they need it, seeking out more nutritious meals rather than grabbing food on the run or existing on ready-meals. Essentially, you develop an intuitive sense of what is right for your body. There are, nevertheless, plenty of 'rules' written about what you 'can' and 'can't' eat or drink before yoga. Steer clear of cold water, some say, being sure only to drink water at 'room temperature'. Potatoes, suggest others, are bad – while fasting is good.

Although I don't think it's necessary at all when you're starting out (if ever), there's plenty written, too, about matching what you eat to your Ayurvedic dosha. In Indian medicine, individuals are divvied up into three dominant constitutional types, or doshas – pitta, kapha and vata – which can complicate eating and drinking enormously. Let's take that 'cold water' rule: it may not be beneficial for vata types, and can exaggerate digestive problems in kapha types, but pitta people, by contrast, may find that it actually soothes digestion. (I'm pitta, which suggests – accurately – that I'm really bad at skipping meals and fasting.) If you'd like to explore the subject, I've some book recommendations on page 221, but meanwhile, I'd counsel an approach of trying to tune in to what your body is asking you for. (And truly, after a while, it will move on from chocolate to other food groups.)

The one universal rule that does hold true with yoga, however, seems to be not to eat before your practice. Most people find it's best not to eat for at least three hours or so beforehand, to allow for digestion. (Some would advise not eating the night before, if you've scheduled an early class – but I for one would find myself collapsing in Downward Dog if I went without food for that long, see the pitta observation above). Most of us find this out the hard way, with the croissant we grabbed en route to class making life extremely uncomfortable for the hour or so we're on the mat, when we find ourselves distracted by digestive rumblings and mumblings, or by brunch 'repeating' on us as we twist, bend and attempt inversions. Everyone's different, though, so you'll have to make that important link for yourself: ask, 'What's the best time for me to eat, before a class, to give me energy, but not interfere with my yoga?' And from there, the next logical step is to ask, 'What are the foods that make me feel best, on the mat?'

On the following pages are some suggestions for dishes that work best at sustaining me and my yoga acquaintances before and after yoga sessions and in day-to-day life.

> As you gain a sense of harmony and balance you may well find that your emotional relationship to food changes – because you are being sustained and energised by yoga

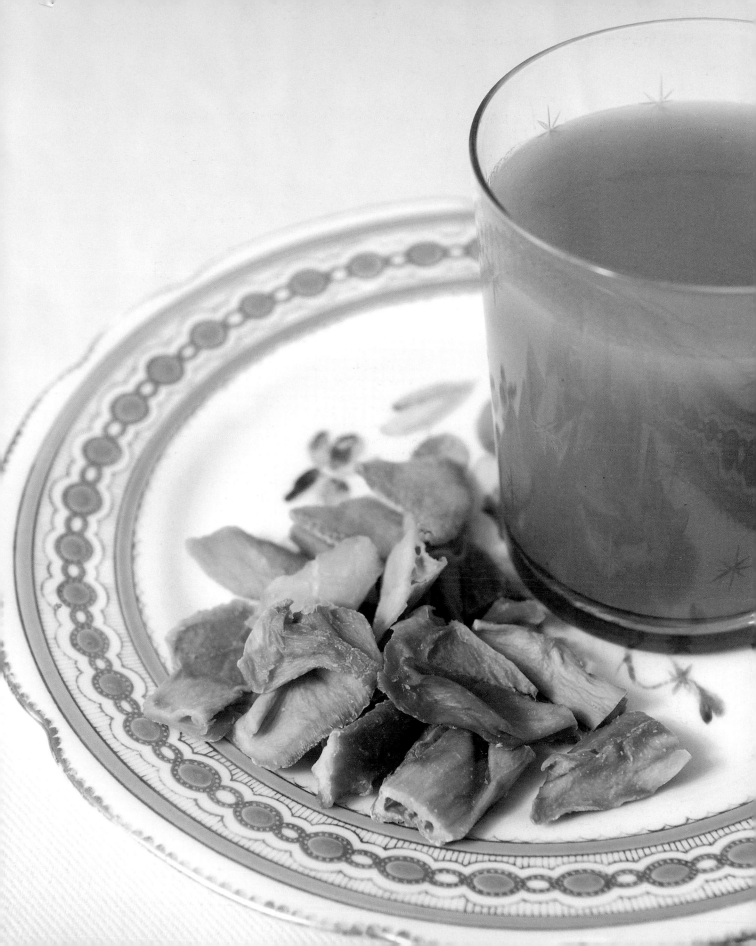

CHAI

Eating before a yoga class or your home practice is a really, really bad idea, no matter how hungry you are. But for me, a cup of chai is a wonderful prelude to a yoga class: a touch of sugar or honey gives a little extra energy and while there's no scientific proof that the warming spices help muscles to relax, that's what it feels like, to me. It's equally fantastic after a yoga session. I like to make decent quantities of chai at a time (this recipe makes about a litre), and I start making it a day in advance; chai keeps well for a couple of days in the fridge (actually, I find it gets better as the spice flavours 'emerge'). It can be heated and reheated perfectly well in a pan on the stove. (Microwaving and yoga seem incompatible, but that might just be me.) If you don't have a spice/coffee grinder, buy ready ground coriander seeds and cardamom (though they won't taste so fresh).

MAKES ABOUT 1 LITRE
1¼ teaspoons coriander seeds
3 tablespoons fresh cardamom pods
½ teaspoon black peppercorns
6cm approx. piece (or 2 x 3cm pieces) of fresh ginger, grated
**   or finely chopped**
1 cinnamon stick
4 cloves
a dash of ground allspice
720ml soya milk, rice milk or cow's milk
2–3 tablespoons black tea
maple syrup, honey or sugar, to sweeten

Using a spice or coffee grinder, whizz the coriander seeds and the cardamom pods into a powder.

Place 280ml of water in a large saucepan and add the peppercorns, ginger, cinnamon stick, cloves and allspice. Bring to the boil, then take off the heat and allow to cool. Refrigerate overnight.

Next day, put the milk in a pan and bring to the boil over a medium heat, stirring continuously and being careful not to scorch it. Add the tea and simmer for 5 minutes. Strain and sweeten to taste with maple syrup, honey or sugar.

CHAI OATMEAL

Chai and yoga just go together; it must be an Indian thing. I was inspired to combine chai with porridge by a recipe from Mollie Katzen's Sunlight Café (Mollie is the renowned author of *Moosewood Cookbook*, one of the all-time best natural food bibles), which adds Ayurvedic spices to hearty breakfast grains. This is a basic recipe to play around with: tinker with the spice levels and add dried fruit such as sultanas and raisins. It tastes amazing on a winter morning after an early yoga practice. Mollie suggests adding a topping of chopped pistachio nuts (yum), but toasted almonds are also utterly delicious.

SERVES ONE HUNGRY PERSON
340ml milk
¼ teaspoon cinnamon
¼ teaspoon ground coriander
¼ teaspoon ground cardamom
¼ teaspoon ground turmeric
¼ teaspoon salt
1–2 drops vanilla extract (optional)
2 teaspoons runny honey
75g rolled oats
2 tablespoons oat bran

Pour the milk into a medium-sized saucepan. Add the spices and the salt, and whisk with a fork to blend them into the milk. Place the pan over a medium heat. Just before the milk comes to the boil, reduce the heat and allow it to simmer for about 5 minutes. Stir in the vanilla extract (if using) and the honey, and whisk again until the honey is dissolved.

Sprinkle in the oats and the oat bran, and stir once or twice. Cover the pan and leave it over a really low heat for around 8 minutes, being sure to stir occasionally to prevent it from sticking. Serve hot.

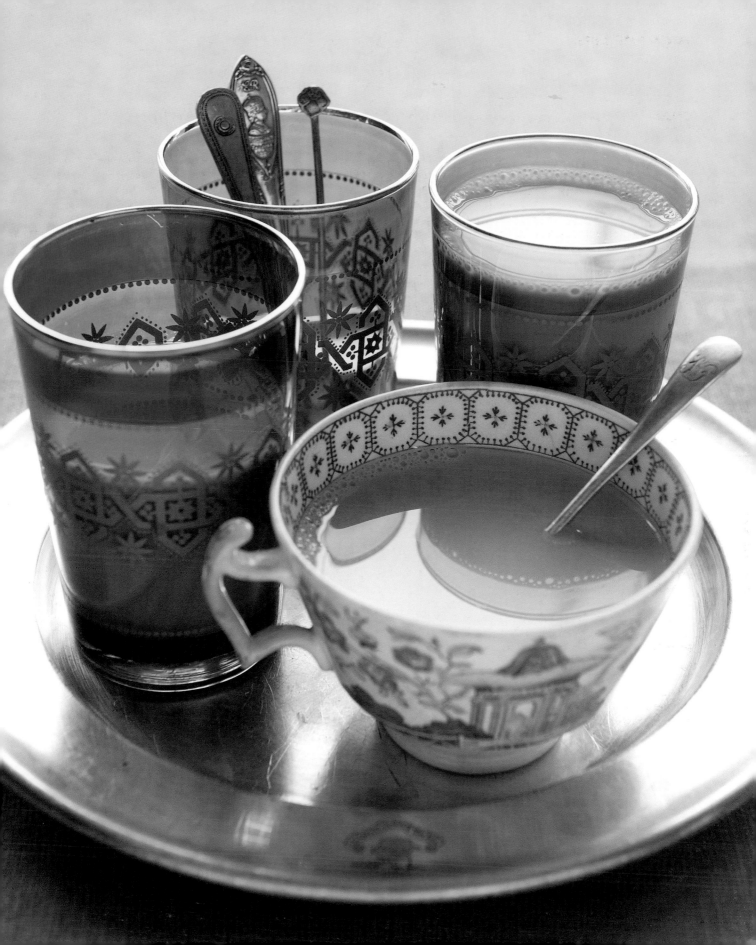

A SUPERBLY SUSTAINING SOUP

Not so much a soup, this is more a meal in a bowl. Barley is a favourite ingredient in Eastern Europe, and though it is less popular elsewhere, it is a fantastically nourishing grain, found easily in natural food stores. I have a love/hate relationship with both celery and fennel, and sometimes they just don't appeal, so the soup works just fine if you leave them out. Like many soups, this tastes even better next day (and the day after...).

SERVES 6
150g medium pearl barley
2.4 litres vegetable stock (see recipe, right, or make using
   Marigold Swiss Vegetable Bouillon Powder)
3 tablespoons olive oil
165g chopped onion or shallots
75g carrots, chopped
75g mushrooms (any type of fresh mushroom is fine, or soak
   dried shiitake or porcini mushrooms and measure when
   they've plumped up), finely sliced
50g celery or fennel, chopped
salt and freshly ground black pepper, to taste
110ml dry sherry (optional)
a few sprigs of chopped fresh parsley, to garnish

Rinse the barley (it's best to do this with any grain) and place it in a large saucepan with three cups of the stock. Place over a medium heat. If you're using homemade stock, add a pinch of salt; if you're using stock made from bouillon powder, it may be salty enough already. Bring the stock to the boil, turn the heat down to a simmer and cover the pan. The liquid should be absorbed within an hour (check occasionally so that the pan doesn't boil dry). Remove from the heat and use a fork to fluff up the grain.

While the grain is cooking, in a large saucepan heat the olive oil over a medium heat, then add the onions or shallots, carrots, mushrooms and celery or fennel. Stir the vegetables constantly for a few minutes, until they have softened. Then add the remaining stock, salt and pepper (taste at this point to adjust the flavour), and bring to a boil. Once the soup has reached boiling point, cover the pan, reduce the heat and simmer for around half an hour.

Now add the cooked barley. If you like a richer flavour, add the sherry, which makes a nice flourish and rounds out the flavours; simmer for a few more minutes so that the alcohol evaporates. Taste again, adjust the seasoning, then throw on the parsley, to prettify, just before serving.

VEGETABLE STOCK

This makes a good base for any soup (see left) and for the vegetable stew on page 184. Feel free to use other raw vegetables you may have around: broccoli, a cabbage leaf or two, fennel, mushrooms, leeks. The principles are the same, even if the final stock tastes subtly different.

MAKES ABOUT 2 LITRES
2 carrots, peeled and roughly chopped
2 celery stalks, roughly chopped
2 onions, peeled and quartered
a handful of parsley
6 black peppercorns
1 dried bay leaf

Put everything into a large saucepan and cover with 2 litres of cold water. Cover with a lid, bring to the boil over a medium heat, then reduce the heat and allow to simmer for 30 minutes. Strain, discarding the vegetables, and the stock is ready for using to make soups and other dishes.

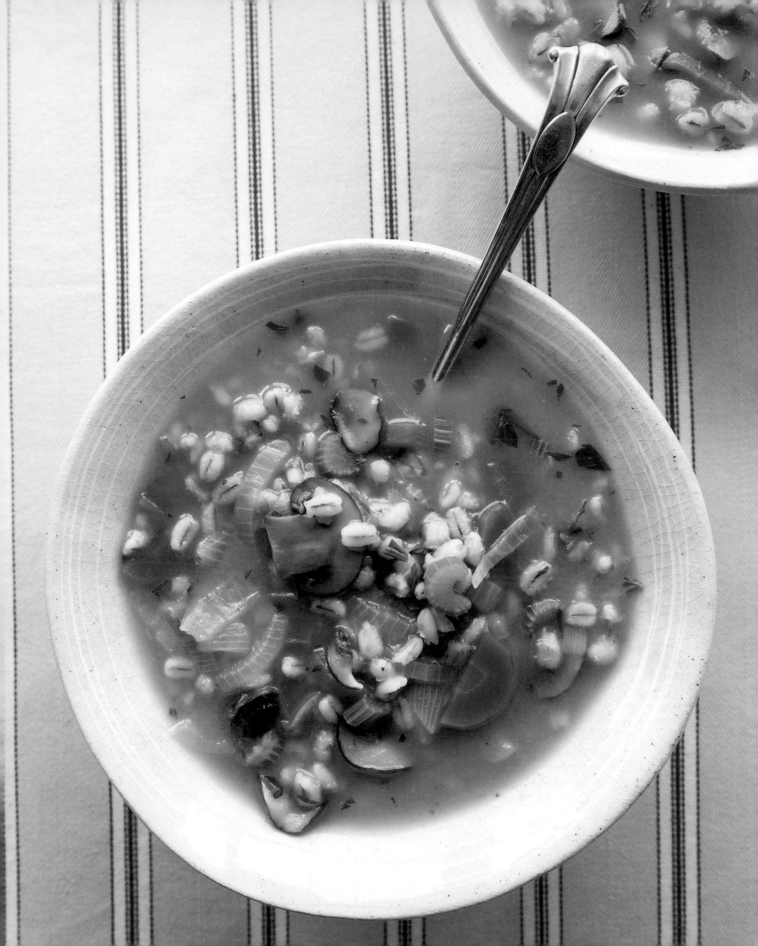

RICE AND GREENS

With seasonal variations, this simple stir-fry is fundamental to my life; it's a recipe that my husband Craig Sams wrote down for his book *The Macrobiotic Brown Rice Cookbook*, and we eat it (or something like it) pretty much every night. Once you've mastered the basic recipe, the potential for the aforementioned variations is huge: add peas, sweetcorn, purple-sprouting broccoli and leaves including dandelions, cauliflower leaves, radicchio, curly endive and flat parsley. For more variations, add herbs generously – fresh marjoram goes well, or try fresh dill or fennel. Or sprinkle Japanese wasabi powder into the dish, to give it more bite. Serve with a light sesame tahini and soya sauce on the side (and maybe a salad, during the summer months) for a highly nutritious meal, which I find very 'grounding' and energy-boosting. The main focus in this recipe is on green vegetables, which are rich in vitamin A, boost the immune system and also help prevent anaemia. That's why this dish is terrific as part of a vegetarian diet.

SERVES 4 (AS A SIDE DISH), OR FEWER (IF MAIN DISH)
3 tablespoons roasted sesame oil
½ onion, peeled and sliced
2 garlic cloves, chopped
8 spring onions
450g greens, sliced into strips
1 teaspoon chopped fresh ginger
750g cooked brown rice
1 teaspoon grated lemon zest (optional if you're rushed)
1 teaspoon lemon juice
soy sauce, to taste
sea salt, to taste

In a large saucepan, warm the sesame oil over a medium heat, then sauté the onion, garlic and spring onions for a few minutes. Add the greens and ginger and stir-fry for another few minutes, until soft. Stir in the rice, lemon zest (if using) and lemon juice, and combine well. Season to taste with soy sauce and salt.

Add enough water to cover the bottom of the pan (about half a cup). Cover the pan with a lid and gently simmer until the water is absorbed, about five minutes. Serve immediately.

What frequently happens, I've observed, is that people start to recognise what food their body actually needs, and when they need it, seeking out more nutritious meals rather than grabbing food on the run or existing on ready-meals. Essentially, you develop an intuitive sense of what is right for your body

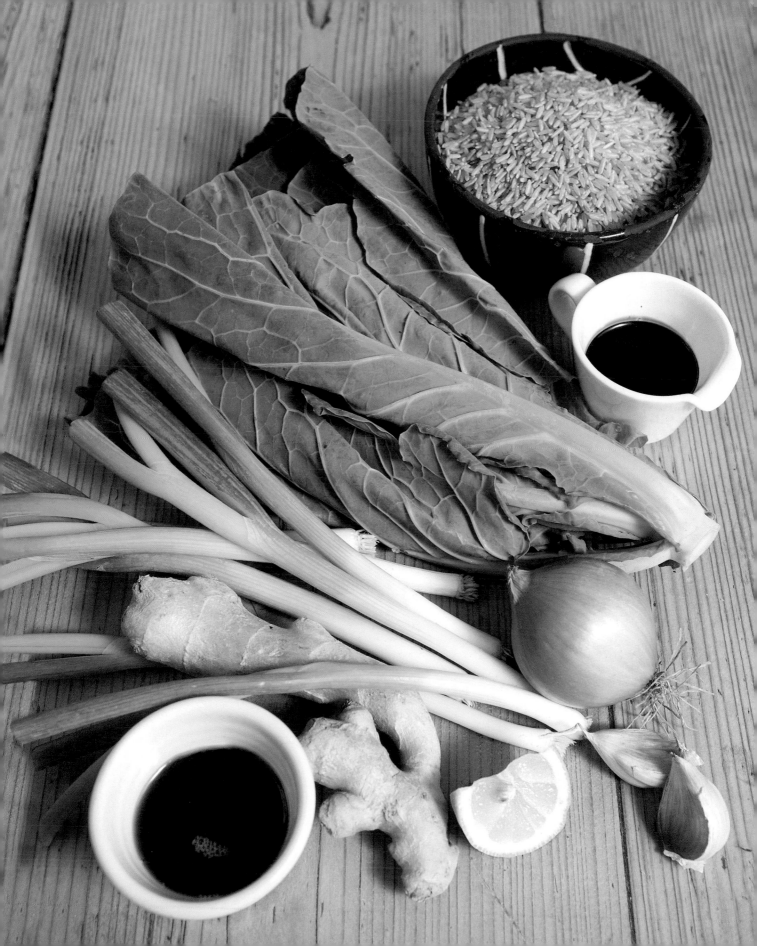

KERALAN VEGETABLE STEW

Kerala in South India is home to many Ayurvedic yoga retreats, and this is a typical, sustaining, lightly spiced Keralan curry which – like the Rice and Greens on page 182 – you could basically live on. So I suggest scaling up the recipe to make generous quantities that you can freeze or keep in the fridge for future meals, liberating yourself from time at the stove – which you can spend on the mat, instead, if you choose. You can use any kind of vegetables, just avoid strongly coloured varieties, such as beetroot, which will taint the colour of the dish. Serve with rice or Indian bread (such as chapattis or naan).

SERVES 4
350g chopped vegetables (carrots, any kind of green beans, potatoes, courgettes, marrow, onions, peas)
1 teaspoon peanut oil or sunflower oil
4 cardamom pods
a few peppercorns
1 cinnamon stick
2 dried bay leaves, slightly crushed
1 large piece of fresh ginger (the size of a couple of fingers), peeled and grated, or cut into small chunks
480ml vegetable stock (see recipe, page 180, or make using Marigold Swiss Vegetable Bouillon Powder)
480ml coconut milk
1 teaspoon lemon juice

Parboil the vegetables and reserve the water you cooked them in to use as stock.

Heat the oil in a large heavy-bottomed pan. Add all the spices to the pan (including the bay leaves) and stir-fry for a minute or two, until they release their flavour. Then add the ginger and continue frying for a few more minutes. Add the parboiled vegetables and sauté for 2–3 minutes.

Pour in the vegetable stock (using the reserved cooking water as part of it), the coconut milk and lemon juice, and cook over a high heat for 10 minutes, then reduce the heat and simmer until the vegetables are done. Serve immediately.

Start making the way you eat more yogic by setting yourself this challenge. Ask yourself, 'What did I last eat? What did it taste or smell of? Did I really enjoy it?'

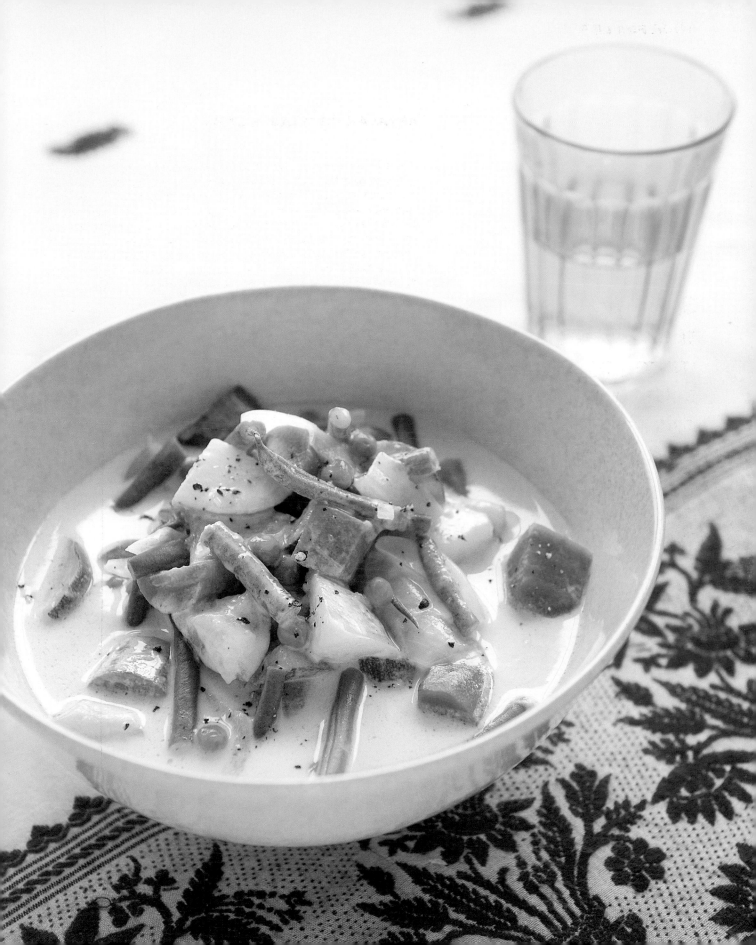

PERFECT PEARS

Traditionally, pears are poached in a sugary syrup, which can play havoc with blood-sugar levels. And as you get deeper into your yoga, I will bet that this is something that you will, increasingly, choose to avoid. This version uses fruit juice for poaching instead. It works best with ripe, firm pears; for softer pears, you may be able to halve the cooking time but to me, this dessert is then a bit squishy. Serve with a dollop of Greek or plain/vanilla-flavored soya yogurt.

SERVES 3
3 pears, sliced in half
480ml cranberry juice
2 cinnamon sticks
4 cloves
a few fresh mint leaves, to garnish

Peel the pears with a paring knife and scoop out the seeds using a teaspoon. Place the pears in a large saucepan over a medium heat, with the fruit juice, the cinnamon sticks and the cloves. Be sure that the juice perfectly covers the pears, and allow to simmer until soft (15 minutes for firm pears; half that for soft pears). Use a fork to test for doneness; it should enter the flesh easily.

Remove the pears from the liquid using a slotted spoon and let them cool on a plate. Then reduce the heat and simmer the poaching liquid for 40–45 minutes, until it is reduced to about a third of the original liquid and is thick and syrupy. Remove from the heat.

Place the pears on a plate flat-side down, and drizzle with the syrup; dress them up with a mint leaf, to serve. They can be enjoyed hot or cold.

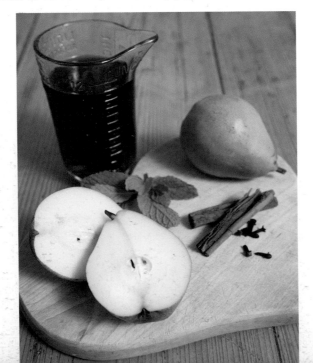

SPICED BAKED APPLES

I'm not saying that dessert is off the menu for yogis, but once you start 'honouring' your body with a yoga practice, it just seems natural to steer clear of junk, especially refined sugars which can send your blood-sugar levels on something of a rollercoaster ride. Dates and sultanas add sweetness to these apples, while the spices are almost aromatherapeutically comforting. Do use cooking apples, which hold their shape and texture better than eating apples. If you like something creamy with your fruit, try a scoop of unsweetened Greek yogurt or soya yogurt.

SERVES 4
4 large cooking apples
6 pitted dates
100g sultanas or raisins, soaked
 in water to plump them up
1 teaspoon ground cinnamon
a shaving or pinch of nutmeg

Preheat the oven to 180°C/gas mark 4. Wash and core the apples, leaving 1cm or so at the bottom of each apple, to contain the fruit filling.

Chop the dates and combine them with the soaked sultanas or raisins, then mix in the spices. Stuff this filling into the apples and place them in a baking dish filled with 5mm of hot water. Bake until the apples are tender, which generally takes 40–60 minutes, then serve hot or cold.

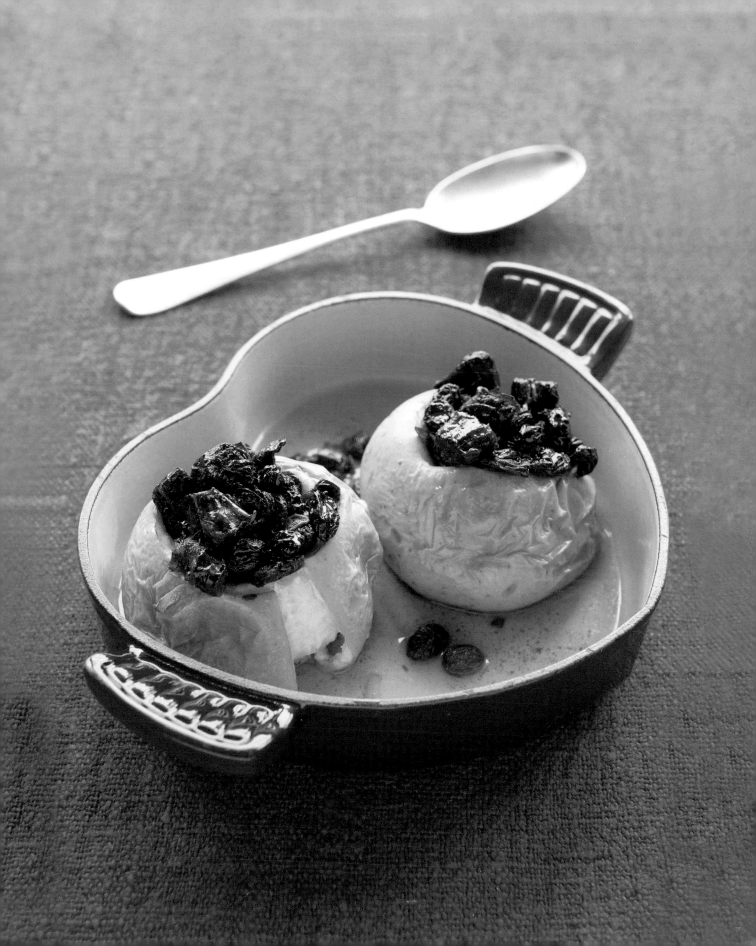

Mindful eating seems to go beautifully hand in hand with yoga

MINDFUL EATING

Most of us – especially those of us watching our waistlines – have probably grasped by now that we are what we eat. And that eating too many sugary and fatty foods is the fast track to a muffin-top, or worse. But there is now a dawning realisation that when it comes to a healthy weight, it may be better not to change what you eat. After all, 95 per cent of diets fail, according to Elyse Resch, author of *Intuitive Eating: A Revolutionary Programme That Works* (see page 221). Instead, 'mindful eating' (also known as 'intuitive eating') works to change how you eat. And actually, that's much easier.

Research is now confirming that that one key reason we pile on the pounds in this stressful, frantic world – one in which we race between appointments, answer e-mails on the bus and speak to friends on the phone while tidying the living room with the other hand – is because we're just not paying attention to what we put in our mouths. I write this as someone who's probably not the only person in the world to have caught herself munching a bowl of cereal while walking upstairs or making the bed. But quite simply, when we eat mindlessly, the appetite centre in the brain isn't satisfied – it doesn't know when to switch off. As a result, we go on eating long after our bodies need it. The result? An ever tighter waistline, not to mention a raft of health challenges.

Mindful eating seems to go beautifully hand in hand with yoga, the mindful practice of moving and breathing. So start making the way you eat more yogic by setting yourself this challenge. Ask yourself, 'What did I last eat? What did it taste like or smell of? Did I really enjoy it?' The chances are you may not even remember – and you're not alone. The really good news is that by learning to re-focus on what you eat, you will actually turbo-charge your pleasure in eating, too. 'If you look at cultures that have done a better job than ours of maintaining healthy weights, such as Mediterranean countries like France, you'll notice people having desserts and full-fat cheeses – but they're not eating half a pound at a time,' says Michael Zemel, director of the Nutrition Institute at the University of Tennessee. 'They've developed a sense of enjoyment about their food, so that a little bit is enough.' Scientists at the University of Pennsylvania have shown that even at McDonald's, the French eat less and more slowly than the Americans!

Post-yoga snacking

So, you didn't eat before your yoga session, you've just done a practice and are about to keel over from light-headedness. Ideal foods after a yoga workout contain a balance of protein and carbohydrates, which your body can break down into amino acids to help repair muscles and boost your energy. It can be helpful to carry a little bag of mixed nuts and dried fruits (a.k.a. 'trail mix') as a post-yoga bite. Alternatively go for an energy bar (check it's not packed with sugar, which plenty are), porridge (see recipe, page 178), soup (see recipe, page 180) or a protein shake: all light, yet containing easily digestible protein. Georgia Wolfenden of www.glowgetter.co.uk swears by The Synergy Company's Pure Synergy (see page 221), a 'green food' powder which is also delicious zooshed up with soya milk (and perhaps a banana), and delivers a potent blend of phytonutrients – from algae, sea vegetables, spinach, kale and berries – which are also fantastic for the skin.

Never eat except at a table,
with cutlery and a plate

There's a famous saying that every journey begins with a single step – and that's certainly true of mindful eating. So, starting with your very next meal, just decide to eat more mindfully. It's as easy as paying attention to these few basics:

Tune into your hunger before you eat

Dr. Ronna Kabatznick, a leading advocate of mindful eating who introduced 'mindful awareness' to the WeightWatchers® programme, says, 'It can help you decide how much food you need, rather than how much you want – and understand why you're eating in the first place. Are you stressed? Happy? Tired? Worried? Is it just because it's lunchtime? Or are you really, truly hungry?' The last question is the only one that truly counts. If you're stressed or worried, do a yoga pose or two or some stretches, or take four drops of Bach Rescue® Remedy if you're really anxious. But don't hit the biscuit tin, which is the first line of action for many people. Sometimes, when you think you're hungry, you're actually thirsty – so try a glass of water before eating, and see if that satisfies you.

Never eat except at a table, with a knife and fork and a plate

Balancing a plate (or worse, a pizza carton) on your lap is the very worst thing you can do in terms of mindfulness: you go on devouring those slices while watching your favourite show, and before you know it, the box is empty. Try to make an effort to lay a table prettily, with proper cloth napkins (use napkin rings to save on washing), flowers, nice plates and even silver (it's incredibly cheap to source at boot fairs or yard sales and doesn't need polishing as often as you'd think!). All this helps to turn every meal into a special event – and your brain notices that.

Get out a tape measure and measure your plates

Research has shown that the ideal size for a plate is 22–25cm. Any smaller and you'll be going back for seconds; bigger, and you'll pile on more to begin with. According to Brian Wansink, PhD, author of *Mindless Eating: Why We Eat More Than We Think* (see page 221), downsizing from a 30cm to a 25cm plate encourages people to eat 22 per cent less.

Make sure the room isn't too bright or noisy

Or, conversely, too dark and quiet. Being over-stimulated can trigger over-eating – but if the atmosphere is too low-key, you may actually linger for too long at the table. If you're alone and you really can't face a meal in silence, put on some soothing classical music.

Make yourself something you really enjoy

Food needn't be complicated, but it does need to stimulate all the senses – including sight. Before starting to eat, look at the food on your plate: notice the colours and the textures before you pick up your knife and fork.

Relax before you eat

If you find it helps, say a silent grace; something to make you appreciate the food in front of you, maybe thanking the many people who grew the ingredients and oversaw their journey to your plate. Take a few deep, slow breaths to still yourself. And never eat when you're angry or feeling het up, since heightened emotions will over-ride awareness of what you're eating, and may interfere with digestion, too.

Take serving bowls off the table

Before you pick up your knife and fork remove all serving dishes from the table except bowls containing vegetables (take the spuds off, too, though!). There's then less temptation to re-load your plate, and if you have to get up from the table for seconds, it gives you time to reflect on whether you really do need that extra salad, crumble or stew. Use a small serving spoon, too: in one study (from Cornell University), participants ate 11 per cent less ice cream when using a petite scoop. Another tip: in much the same way, it can be really helpful to keep 'treats' and the foods you find irresistible out of reach. A study carried out by Dr. Wansink (see how much research is going into this area?) showed that female secretaries ate 5.6 times more chocolates if they were placed on a nearby desk than if they had to stand up and walk a mere two metres to get to them!

Focus on every mouthful

When you first put food in your mouth, don't do anything for a moment or two – just savour it on your tongue, and allow the flavours to emerge. Then chew thoroughly and slowly before swallowing. Do the same with every mouthful. A macrobiotic diet is far more restrictive than mindful eating, and asks followers to chew each mouthful 50 times. This helps hugely with digestion, as well as sending messages to your brain that it's really eating something.

Research has shown that the ideal size for a plate is 22–25cm

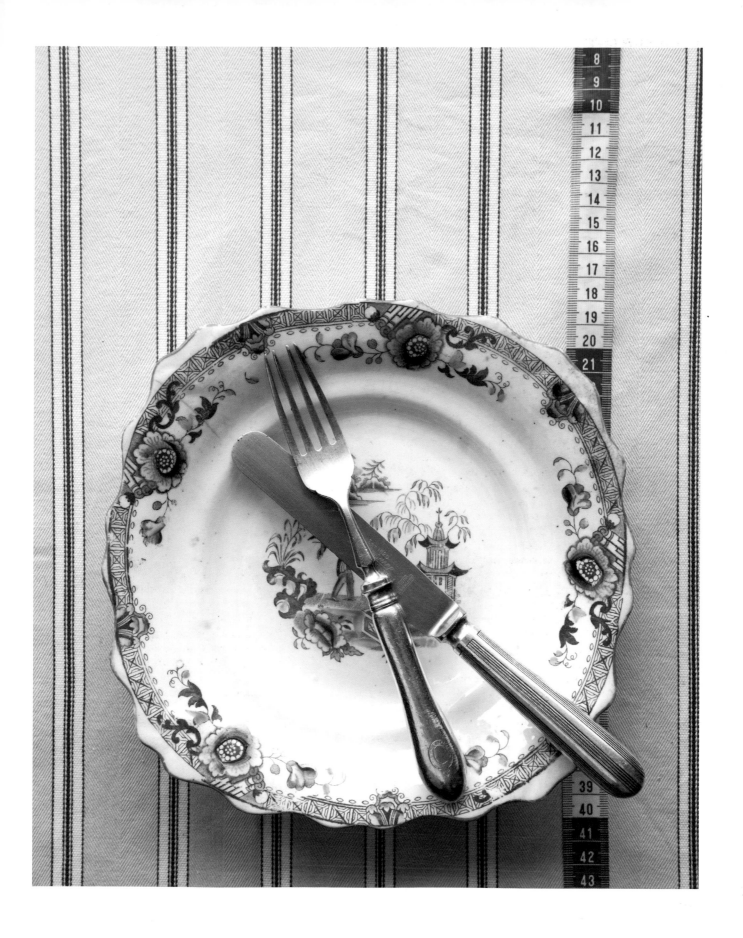

Refocus at several points during the meal

Jean Kristeller, PhD, who runs the Mindfulness-Based Eating Awareness Training Program at Indiana State University, advises, 'Pause for a few moments to refocus on the experience of eating and your sense of satiety.' This gives you an opportunity to think about how much you're eating, but also gives your body (and mind) time to register the sensation of fullness, a physiological process that can take up to 20 minutes.

Let your glasses trick your mind

Drink alcohol from a tall, skinny glass; the mind perceives height more readily than width, so you'll be fooled into thinking you've had more. Apparently, when asked to try pouring the same measures of liquid into short, wide tumblers and tall, thin glasses, we tend to pour at least a quarter more into the short tumblers. So drink water out of short tumblers, and wine from tall ones.

Don't abandon hope (and good habits) when eating out

It's true that 'The biggest challenge to mindfulness is eating with other people,' acknowledges Dr. Ronna Kabatznick. Research has confirmed that humans eat faster and for longer when in larger groups: there seems to be some primitive group-feeding response (if you don't get to the mammoth stew first, someone else will eat it!). What's more, Kabatznick admits, 'Conversation is distracting. But every time you lose your focus or over-eat, just begin again. Every bite, every meal, is a chance to start over...'

And if you do overeat, be kind to yourself

Last but not least, practise the yoga quality of acceptance. If you do over-eat, don't punish yourself by depriving or starving yourself next day, just accept that we're all human – and move on. This way, you should soon find that you really can finally lose weight, drop a dress size and feel lighter one mindful mouthful at a time...

It's perfectly possible to get all of the nutrition you need for a healthy body and balanced mind from vegetable and grain sources

Happier Meals?

Yoga has been found to be helpful for those with full-blown eating disorders. In the US, a clinical psychologist – Lisa Kaley-Isley – who is also a registered yoga teacher, began offering yoga classes to patients with eating disorders. She observes, 'Yoga addresses the mind – where the anxiety and compulsions are – and the body that is the focus of the anxiety and compulsion. It does so with an emphasis on creating strength and flexibility in both.'

Interestingly, a study into 139 women by a researcher at the Preventive Medicine Institute in Sausalito, California, revealed that women who practised yoga felt more positive about their bodies and had healthier attitudes towards food than women, for instance, who did aerobics or ran.

If you overeat, don't punish yourself by depriving or starving yourself the next day – just accept we're all human

THE VEGGIE YOGI

I know there are carnivores who'll read this book and throw it across the room when they get to this paragraph, because I'm about to suggest that yoga might – just might – encourage you to eat less meat, or even give it up entirely. You absolutely do not have to be (or become) a vegetarian to do yoga, but you may become aware – as you start to create links between what you eat and how you feel – that meat makes you feel 'heavy'.

By contrast, eating vegetarian foods – so long as you go easy on the fried spring rolls and the cheese dishes, which can pile on the pounds – can help to maintain the light and energised feeling you get from practising yoga.

And if you want to get into the more spiritual, consciousness-raising side of yoga – rather than doing it for your bad back or because you yearn for Madonna-esque abs – then you may like to take on board the idea of ahimsa, which basically means 'non-harming', and encourages feelings of love and compassion for all living creatures, including animals. Many people who practise yoga reach a point where eating animals just doesn't fit with that.

I'm not saying that if you're not already vegetarian this is definitely going to happen to you; just be aware that it may. And also be aware that it is perfectly possible to get all the nutrition you need for a healthy body and a balanced mind from vegetable and grain sources (even dairy is optional). You might like to download a vegetarian food pyramid from the internet (see page 221).

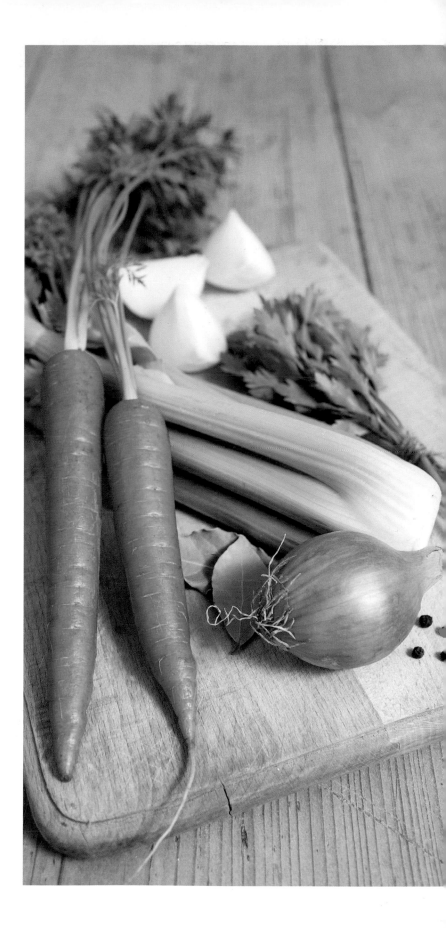

One study revealed
that women who
practised yoga felt
more positive about
their bodies

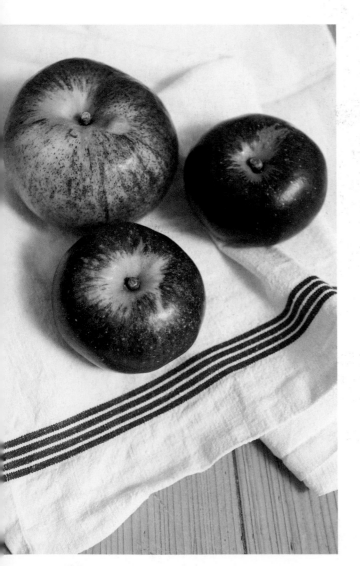

JUICE IT

'Drink your food and chew your drinks.' Whaaaat? Well, this is a phrase that's often used in my house (I am married to the man who introduced macrobiotic foods to Europe...). Essentially, what this simple phrase encourages is chewing your food properly – 50 times per mouthful, if you really want to 'go for it'. But the 'chew your drinks' bit is less easily understood: it means sipping and savouring, not glugging and gulping. One way to enjoy 'chewing' your drinks is to juice at home.

Now, juicing can be a total faff with one of those industrial-quality juicers (which are fiendish to clean, in my experience). A more lifestyle-friendly alternative, I've found, is a high-quality food blender, in which you can easily create a juicy cocktail from just about any fruit and vegetables (ideally, selecting what's in season). Remove stalks (and hard stones or pips) then just zoosh it all up together. The best drinks have a balance of tartness and sweetness – and you can combine flavours just as you would in recipes for solid foods. Melon, mint, strawberries, peaches, blueberries and lemon, for example, make a fruit salad in a glass. While kale, celery, garlic (not to mention wild garlic leaves), chilli, lemon and tomatoes create a sensational 'virgin Mary'. The tomatoes are really not the done thing, macrobiotically – members of the nightshade family, they are said to be bad for joints. But while – like most people – I've made many compromises in my marriage, tomatoes are non-negotiable.

A more low-tech and low-cost juicing option is to push ripe fruit through a fine-mesh strainer, to purée the flesh. But however you juice, the phytonutrients, or plant chemicals, in these fresh, raw foods are easily and swiftly made available to replenish and nourish your body.

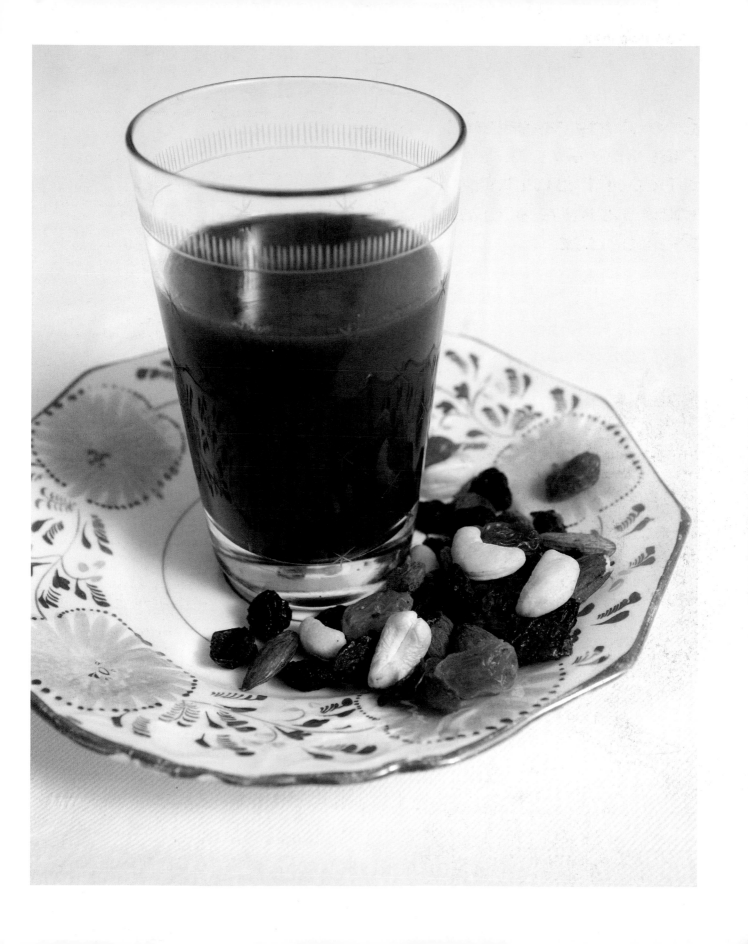

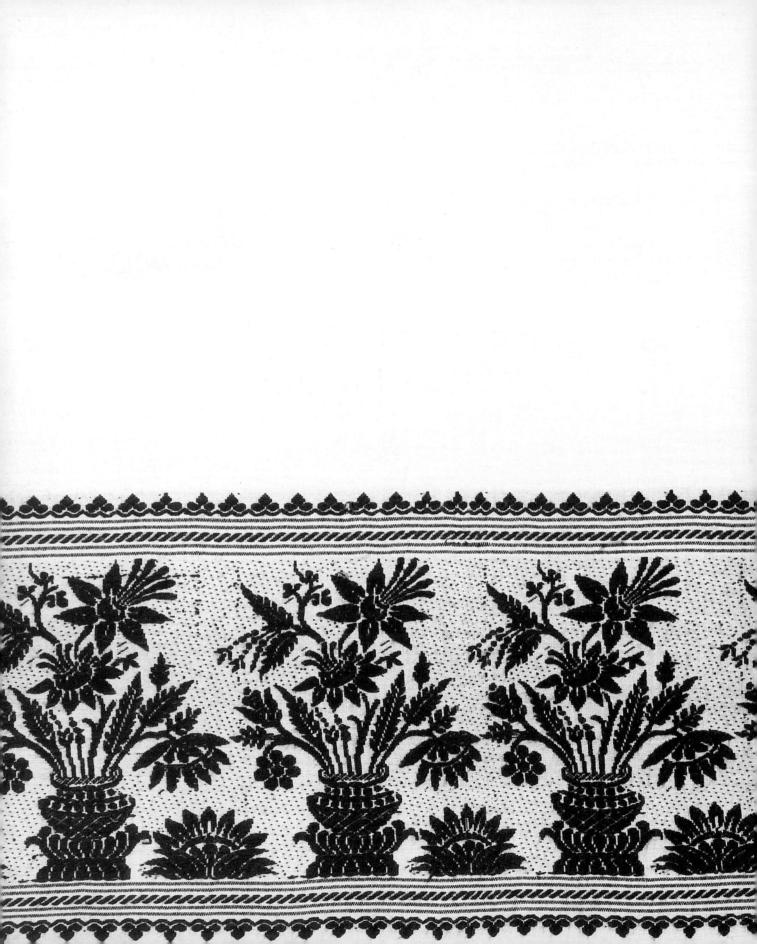

CHAPTER TWELVE

REGAIN YOUR YOGA MOJO

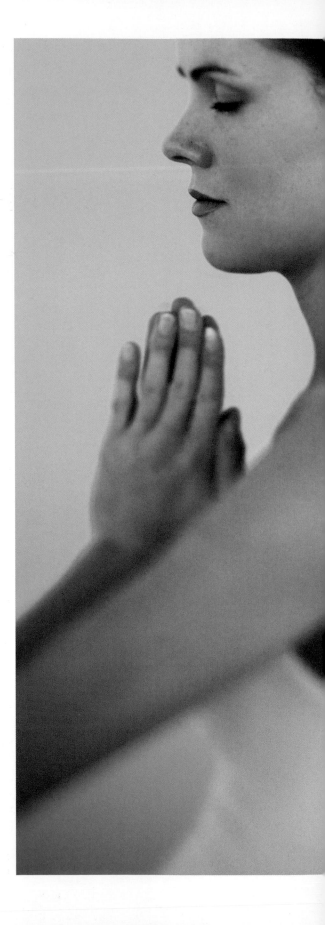

Life is full of responsibilities: keeping people and pets fed, meeting deadlines, taking care of friends and family who are less-than-well or lonely. Motherhood, in particular, is all about putting other people's needs before your own. However, let's think back again to that sage in-flight safety advice – about pulling on your own oxygen mask before putting one on a child. If we don't take care of ourselves, we can't support those around us. It's that simple – and it's that rationale which can encourage us to carve time out of a busy schedule for yoga at home or in a class setting.

If you've ever been on a diet, you'll know what it's like occasionally to lapse. There's generally a lot of self-reproach, sometimes a feeling you've 'blown it', so what-the-hell, why not head straight for the biscuit barrel? It can be the same with yoga, especially in the early days when your body's not necessarily panting for it like a dog with a lead in its mouth. Which is how practising yoga feels for me, making it extremely hard not to spend time on the mat, frankly. But believe me, it took time to get to that place, and it will probably take you time, too.

I've heard the phrase 'yoga blues' to describe how we sometimes find our interest waning. There's often a good reason, and since yoga is partly about self-enquiry, when this happens it's a cue to tap into what that reason might be. Maybe you're bored with your routine and it feels stale. Perhaps your life has changed (less time on your hands, more time on your hands, perhaps a child has left home, leaving you feeling bereft), and you haven't adjusted your practice to fit. Maybe you've just 'hit a wall' physically and don't feel like you're getting anywhere. Generally, it's frowned on to use the phrase 'getting better at yoga', but if you're not any closer to touching your toes...well, we all hear you.

So all is not lost if you miss some classes, or can't seem to dust off the mat that's staring at you from the corner of your office or your practice space at home. Everyone, even Bikram for all I know, has 'yoga slumps' every now and then. We get derailed by illness, injury or just Stuff That Happens, and before we know it realise that we've only practised once in the last month. Ironically, when we think we don't have time for yoga is often when it can help us most, by steadying the mind, clarifying thoughts and delivering the physical strength to deal with a particularly challenging situation.

In meditation, when the mind wanders (as it always does, to all of us), we're encouraged simply to refocus and begin again. It should be the same with yoga. If you fall away from your practice, just come back again. Here are some practical ideas to get you over the slump and regain that discipline.

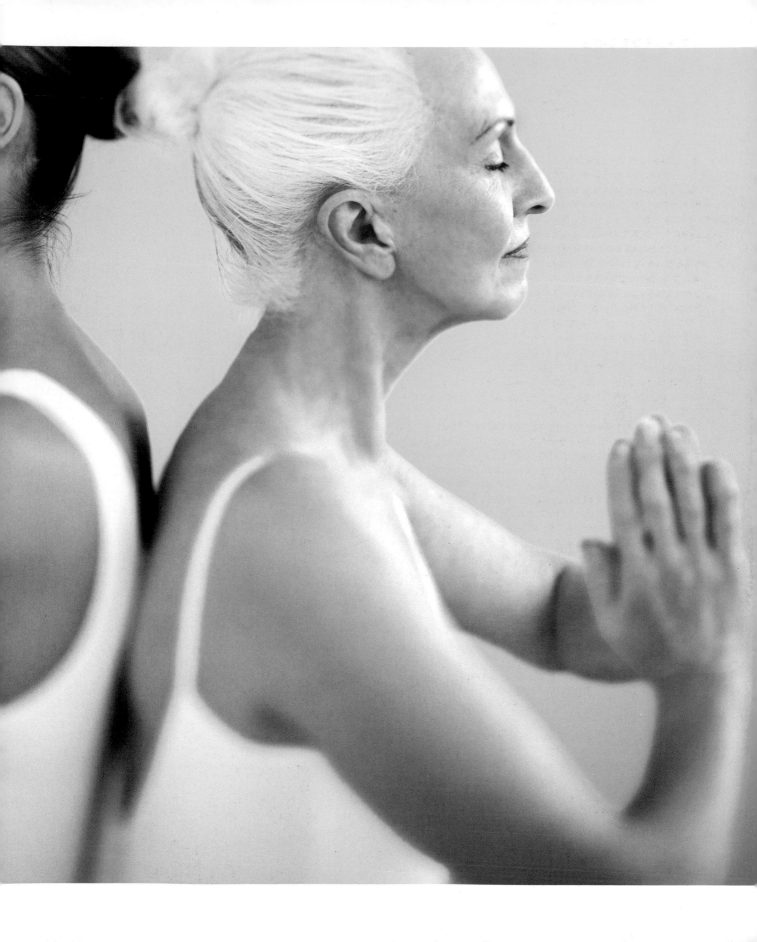

Reward yourself with your favourite postures If you're practising at home, you can coax yourself back into a regular practice with the moves you love most. If it was me, I'd go for Downward-facing Dog Pose, Wide-legged Forward Bend, Two-legged Reclining Twist, Child Pose and (no, it's not necessarily cheating) Corpse Pose. That's far, far better than doing nothing at all, and when you feel energised (and, yes, less guilty) after doing these, you'll almost certainly find yourself ready to move on to more difficult poses.

Set manageable goals Five, ten or 15 minutes of yoga a day can be all you need to get you back into yoga, provided you stick to it regularly. Even if you simply lie on your mat and breathe deeply, it's enough to get you in the 'yoga zone'. If you've been through a phase of several classes a week and it's bothering you that you can't get there that often, drop into class once a week, and pat yourself on the back for making it. Write down your commitment in your diary, or tell a friend/partner that's what you've committed to do, if that helps to reinforce your intention.

Try a different class Maybe boredom is stopping you from going to class. Maybe you feel as if you'll scream if you have to work through that exact same sequence one more time. (That's not exactly the state of mental acceptance that yoga is supposed to inspire, but we're all human.) Checking out a new teacher or a new centre in a different part of town can be a great way to get your yoga mojo back. If you always do yoga at home, get out and experience for yourself what other people do. Although a familiar sequence can be comforting and cocooning during troubled times, when we're feeling stronger variety is truly the spice of yoga life.

Maybe try a beginners' class If you're finding your regular class challenging, be kind to yourself and take the effort down a notch or two. You can catch up and enjoy the practice instead of feeling like you're being over-challenged, and that can be enough to restore your confidence.

Get over the idea that you're 'too busy' Plenty of busy people find time for yoga. Personally, I have a deal with myself: I am never too busy to do yoga. In fact, I am never too busy not to do yoga, because without it I can't deal with my many and varied responsibilities. On the mornings when I do yoga, I have the clarity to sail smoothly and in a considered way through the challenges of the day. I sometimes feel it's like putting on blinkers in terms of helping my focus.

If your teacher leaves, look for a new one fast My yoga 'breaks' have almost invariably come about when a favourite teacher left town or stopped to start a family. It's really, really easy to get out of the habit of going to class when that happens, so my advice is immediately start looking for an alternative, trying on a few classes and teachers for size, if necessary. Otherwise a week becomes a month becomes a year before you know it.

One way to coax yourself back into a regular practice is to do the poses you love the most

Make yoga 'dates' with a friend If you promise to go to a class with a friend, you won't just let yourself down if you opt out, you'll also let him or her down. (But if your friend cancels, stick with your intention.)

Try a little music, to inspire you On page 54 you'll find recommendations for some fantastic yoga tracks that make the perfect background for yoga at home. Stimulating beats can boost energy, meditative sounds can make you calm, and drums can 'ground' you when you've got a serious case of 'head-frazzle'.

Shake up your regime at home Once you know how to do the different poses, play around with the sequence or the speed of your yoga. Practise deliberately and with real awareness, focusing on your breath and observing how it deepens and strengthens a pose.

Treat yourself to some new props We all love a gadget (even when apparently seeking to live a more minimalist, possession-free life). A yoga belt can help with leg stretching; a big inflatable physio-ball can enable you to sit and find your 'centre', improving your posture; a yoga DVD can open your eyes to a new style of yoga. Don't go mad, but it's true that the act of buying a yoga 'accessory' (of which there are more on pages 50–2) can reinforce your intention to practise.

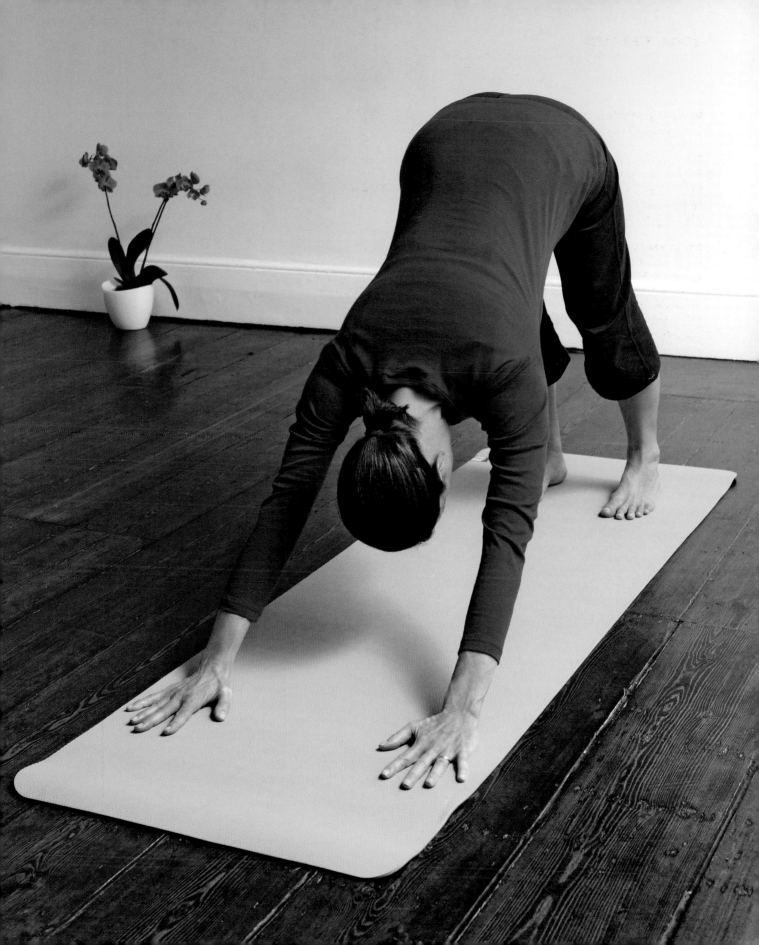

De-junk a bit On pages 46–8, I've made suggestions for creating a 'home space' for yoga. The trouble is, it's often the spare room or a corner that others in your household may not respect the way you do. If that space is getting cluttered with stuff, clear it, then burn some sage and waft it around (this Native American tradition of purification really seems to work). Sweep, dust, vacuum, and generally reclaim that space, making it somewhere you want to unroll your mat again.

Sign up for a yoga conference or workshop These can be great for getting you out of your comfort zone (often the too-comfortable-ness of that zone dulls a passion for yoga), exposing you to new ideas, new teachers and new forms. Open your eyes, widen your horizons and you will almost certainly return to your mat with new commitment.

As with all forms of exercise teaming up with someone else can be very helpful for nudging you to a class

SECRETS OF STICKING TO IT

The real benefits of yoga – a clearer mind, flatter stomach (yes, it really works, even if you feel your abs are basically shot!), better posture and balance – only really come with regular practice. Dropping into a class every now and then is better than nothing, but it's no substitute for daily, or several-times-a-week practice. Here are tried-and-tested tips that can help you stick to it:

Little and often is better than an occasional blitz Try setting aside ten or (better) 15 minutes, either first thing in the morning, when you get home from work (yoga can be a wonderful transition from office to feeling grounded at home) or last thing at night.

Take a yoga break – or two – during the day We tend to hurtle through our days in a frenzy of too-much-to-do-in-too-little-time – and yoga is the ultimate antidote to that. You can set your phone (or any timer) to alert you every couple of hours for a 'yoga break' of mindfulness, and a stretch or two, which will un-kink muscles and de-stress you beautifully. And nobody's going to strike you with a thunderbolt if you 'multi-task' while doing yoga: brushing your teeth in Tree Pose (see page 70), or standing in Mountain Pose (see page 60) while you're waiting for a checkout. This will all help you to feel (and be) more balanced.

Get a 'yoga pal' As with all forms of exercise (which yoga is, in its most basic form), teaming up with someone else can be very helpful for nudging you to a class when it's foul outside. Or take it in turns to visit each other's houses, mat under your arm, and explore a few yoga poses together. You can watch each other, make suggestions, even learn from each other. Maybe you could try a class or workshop that specialises in partner yoga.

Explore individual postures A class, or your home practice, will mostly be a sequence of movements. You may not get the chance to explore each posture very deeply. Try picking a 'posture of the week', promising yourself to do it for a little while each day that week. Go in and out of the pose repeatedly, tapping in to how it makes you feel (physically and emotionally), exploring whether there are ways to make it easier (the right breathing can transform a pose), and generally getting to know it better. I like the saying that you should feel as comfortable in a pose as you do in your favourite pair of jeans.

Variety is the spice of yoga Once you've worked your way through individual poses, you might like to focus on a group of postures: standing, sitting or balancing poses, backbends, whatever. Be guided by your mood and energy levels. Meanwhile, Fridays and the weekend are just perfect for restorative poses.

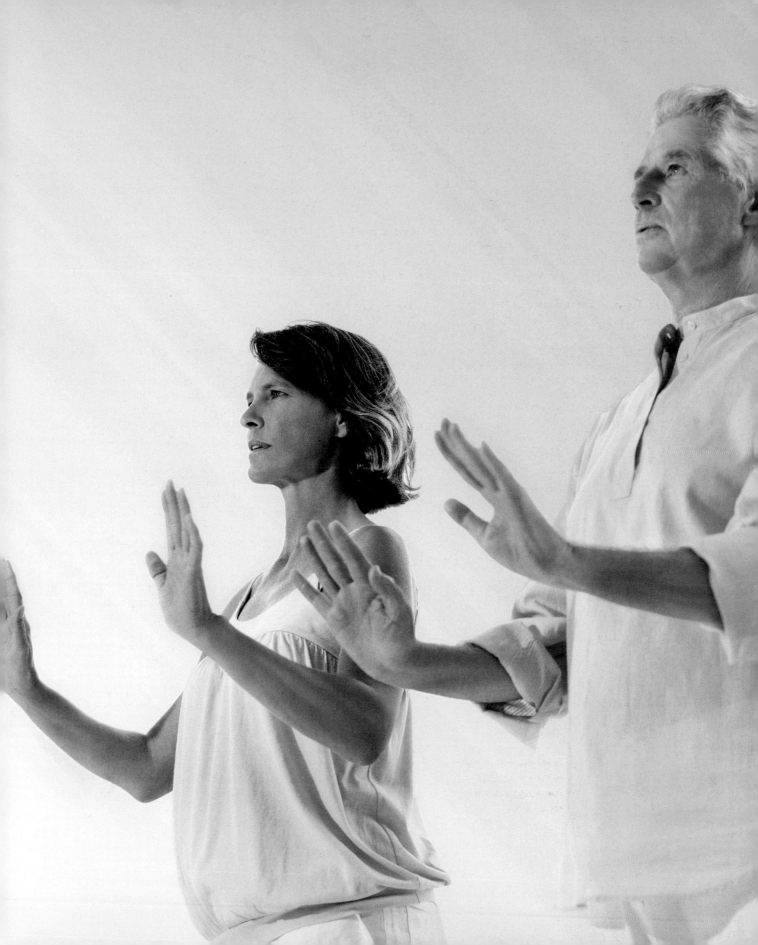

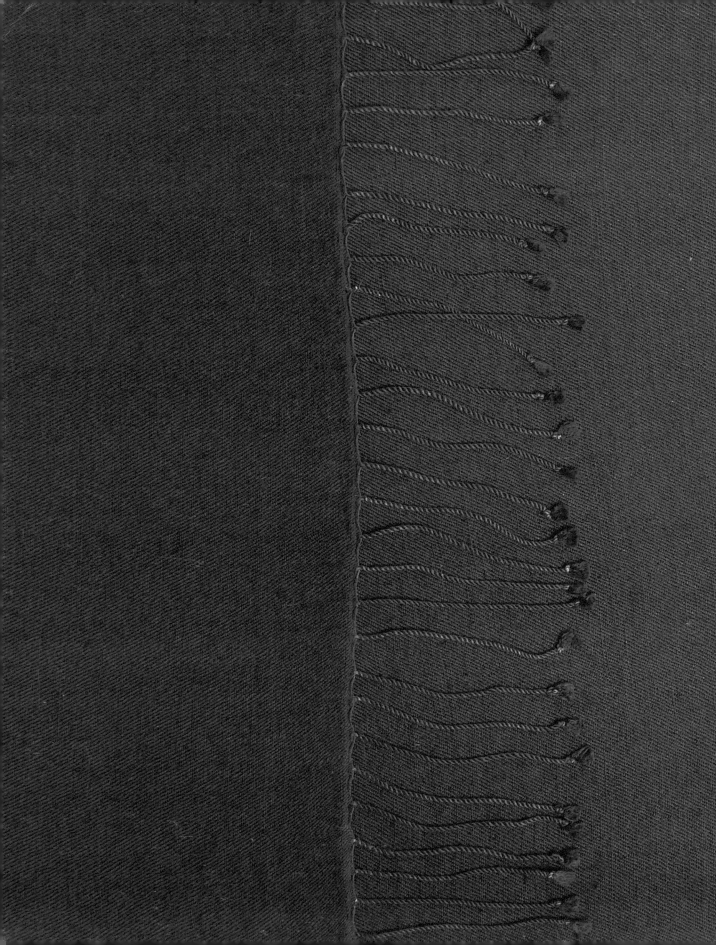

CHAPTER THIRTEEN

HAPPY
(YOGA) HOLIDAYS

M ost of us go on holiday to relax, revive and unwind. Flopping onto a beach with a pile of blockbusters and a piña colada can do that for some people. Others find it reviving to walk the streets of bustling cities, guidebook in hand to track down pitstops for refuelling between visits to museums and monuments.

But for me – and countless other yoga fans – there is quite simply nothing to rival the restorative power of a yoga vacation. I've seen a yoga holiday described as 'not recreation, but re-creation' – and that hits the nail on the head. A yoga vacation can be the ultimate – even life-changing – way to immerse yourself in this pursuit. Sometimes you really have to 'lose' yourself to 'find' yourself....

In my case, the chances of getting my husband on a yoga vacation are about the same as getting him to tightrope across the Grand Canyon (i.e. less than zero), which is good, because in my experience yoga vacations can be fantastic for the lone traveller. Travelling on your own can generally be isolating. But on a yoga vacation, you already have something seriously in common with your fellow travellers: your love of yoga. This makes a great starting point for conversation – and, potentially, for friendship, too. On the other hand, if you 'want to be alone' while on a yoga break, that will be totally respected, too. Maybe you want to meditate. Maybe you want to read a Jackie Collins, sneakily. But you'll usually be left to your own devices, without a fuss, if you choose to spend time on your own.

Not long ago, on a yoga holiday, I met a woman at an all-day workshop who had taken up yoga at the age of 74, after the death of her husband. A decade later, she had friends all over the world who she'd met on her yoga holidays. She was full of laughter and life, and she was more flexible than many people half her age. So it is never too late (and never too early) to treat yourself to a yoga vacation.

Whatever your age and stage in life, though, holidays are precious. So: how can you track down your perfect yoga trip? The usual starting point is to ask friends, as with any other type of trip. So for this chapter I asked two of my friends – who happen to have travelled the world visiting spas, yoga retreats, ashrams and doing classes in far-flung cities – which were their personal favourites. Kathy Phillips, author of *The Spirit of Yoga* (see page 221) and a trained yoga instructor herself, is International Beauty Director for Condé Nast Asia. Former magazine editor Jo Foley (we are frequently mistaken for one another!) has become a highly respected spa 'critic', and is author of *Great Spa Escapes* (see page 221). You'll find their recommendations on the next few pages.

There are some basic guidelines to follow, to get the most out of your yoga holiday, set out on the following pages. But perhaps the most important of them, whether you are getting into yoga or it's already part of your life, is Just Do It. Because you really are worth it!

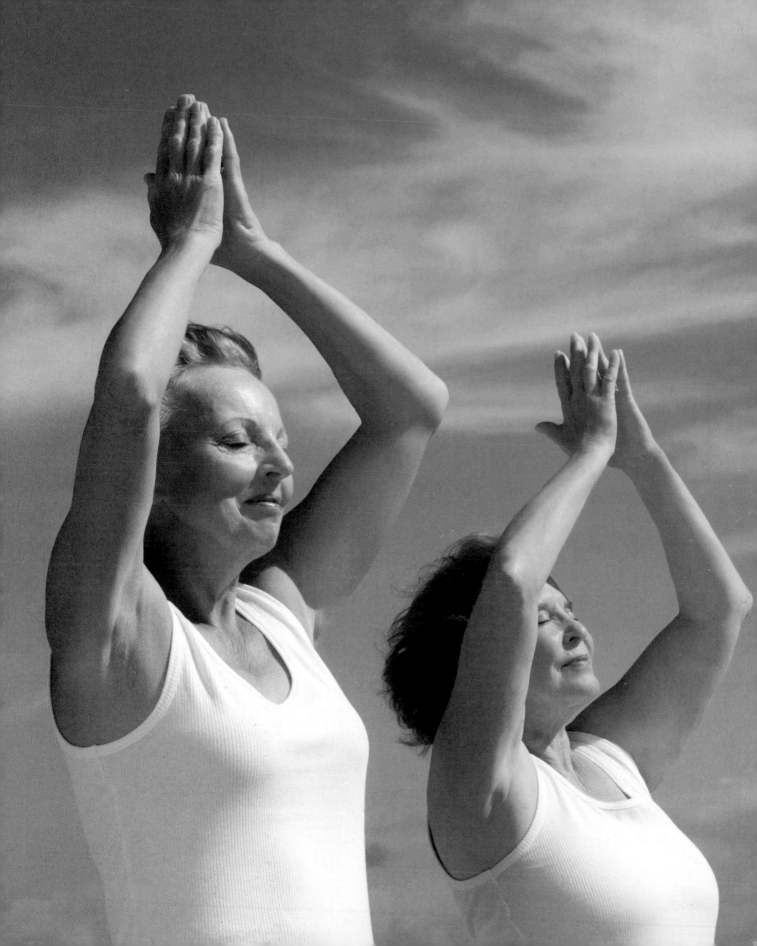

Consider the temperature Selfishly, I'm starting with my No. 1 concern. If you're of *un certain âge*, you may not want to do yoga in the broiling heat. I look on retreat websites to see whether the yoga is done outdoors beneath the blazing sun (that would rule it out for me) and at what time of day. Morning and late afternoon/evening are fine, but I am no Bikram babe and find it seriously challenging to do yoga when it's too hot. The perfect location for me would be a straw-roofed studio, with a cool breeze coming off the sea. There are plenty out there. Alternatively, you may be the sort of person who loves to work up a sweat during yoga, in which case you may adore an outdoor class in the midday sun. But do research these things before you book.

Get the style right If you usually do a gentle form of yoga, you're probably not going to be crazy about a retreat based around power yoga or Astanga – see page 32 for a run-down of these and the many other styles of yoga that may be offered on yoga holidays. If you have a favourite style of yoga, bear that in mind when you plan your great escape. And if your priority is to recover a sense of stillness in a crazy-busy life, look for a vacation that focuses on meditation, or which offers mantra meditation or kirtan chanting. On the other hand, if you're feeling adventurous, you may want to step out of your 'comfort zone' and up the pace on a yoga holiday, using it as a kind of 'taster' for other styles.

Most yoga holidays have a website, and explain what's involved and which style of yoga is taught. If not, feel free to e-mail the organisers before you hit the 'confirm booking' button. When doing this research, you should also get an idea of the schedule: some retreats offer all-day sessions with a break for a (light) lunch; others offer one or two classes at either end of the day. How much yoga do you think you want to do? Don't be over-ambitious is my tip. If you're new-ish to yoga, two daily three-hour sessions may be more than your body can take.

Single, double, dorm? You would not catch me sharing a room with strangers for all the bancha tea in Wholefoods Market. However, you might love bunking up with a couple of (same sex) strangers, or perhaps you're planning a holiday with a friend or group. Naturally, sharing accommodation is less expensive, but most yoga centres do offer some single rooms (these tend to get booked up early, so take that into account when planning your vacation). 'Community' is part of the yoga experience and I'm full of admiration for people who don't mind sharing their space with others. But I'm (happily) married, and having my own room for a week or ten days is rather a treat, giving me time to reflect on my experience.

Find out exactly what's included I'm a pretty seasoned traveller, used to getting from A to B and travelling independently, but even so I always make sure I know before booking what's included in the price. Transfers to and from the yoga location? Taxes and tips? All meals? When you're budgeting, this information is crucial – but it's especially important if you're used to being whisked from airport to destination. Not every yoga holiday does include transfers, and you

wouldn't be the first person to be found sobbing over an erratic Italian bus timetable by the roadside. Never a great start to a vacation.

Other yoga vacations, meanwhile, offer tuition only, leaving you free to organise local accommodation and eat where you want. These less structured packages up the hassle and planning factor, but may save you money.

Research the 'pamper factor' Yoga retreats can be pretty spartan – particularly ashrams and rustic retreats. Others can be more indulgent and may also offer additional massage or pampering treatments, which can help you to unwind still further. Again, take a little time to check out what else is on offer.

What other 'action' is there? Want to combine your yoga with an outdoorsy pursuit such as hiking, kayaking, white-water-rafting – or a more gentle pursuit, such as cooking or watercolour painting? My suggestion is to Google 'yoga and painting holiday' (followed by your 'dream' destination), and see what comes up: you may find your perfect 'combo' of activities. If you're the yoga 'bunny' in a relationship and you'd actually quite like to go away with your (non-yoga-loving) partner, you may find a holiday that offers something for both of you.

Will the food sustain you? As a vegetarian I tend to find that the food on offer at yoga vacations is right up my street; if you're a carnivore, and you feel you need protein for energy, check out what the menu's likely to feature. (Fact: it's easier to find vegetarian yoga retreats than those that do offer meat.) Also get an idea of how many meals a day you'll be offered, and how light they may be: some retreats are more of a 'detox' and it can be hard to get enough to keep you going through classes without feeling faint. That's certainly happened to me, and as someone whose blood sugar is a bit rollercoaster-y, I prefer to eat regularly and have the energy for class, rather than be deprived and keel over. A quick e-mail to the organisers, if the information is unclear,

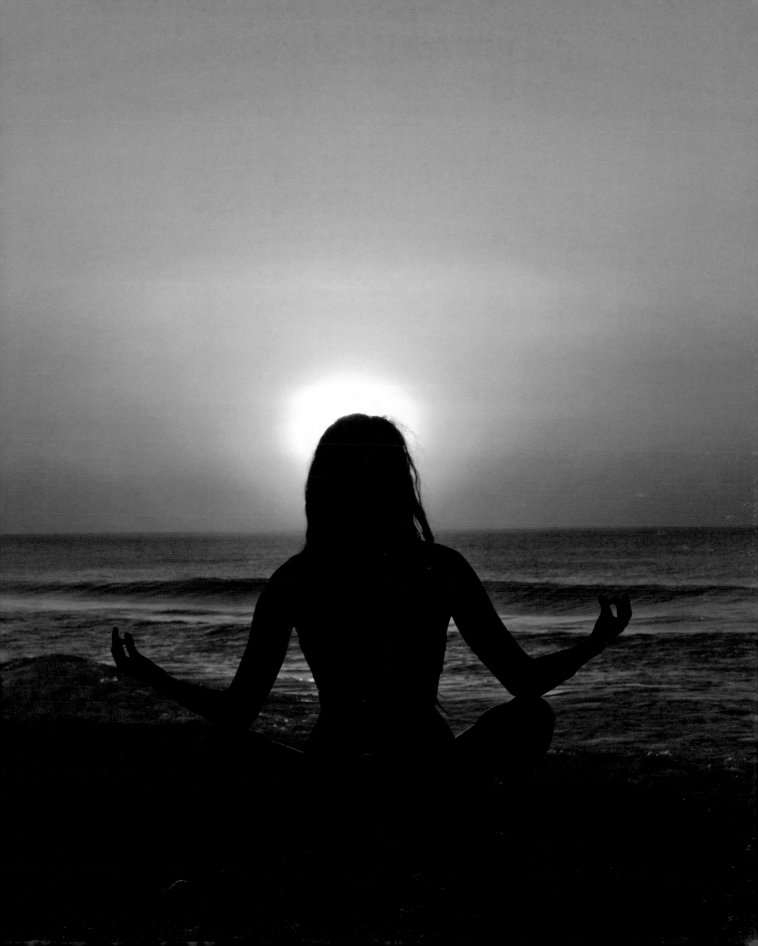

can be helpful. If you have any special dietary requirements, allergies and intolerances, do let the organisers know before you go; most retreats are fantastically accommodating.

Most true yoga retreats are alcohol-free, though you may get a glass of wine on your last night – so bear this in mind if you're a daily-glass-of-wine (or two) sort of person. Caffeine may also be off the menu, so if you're used to coffee or tea throughout the day, you can end up listless and with the most almighty headache. As a tea drinker (if this is my 'worst' vice, I figure I'm doing OK), in the past I've 'negotiated' with the organisers to have a cup of caffeinated tea in the morning, and another at 'tea-time'. I've found from personal experience of going caffeine-free that I just get more out of the experience if I can have a l-i-t-t-l-e bit of English Breakfast. They're generally fine about this. (And the only time they weren't, I have to confess I snuck out to a local café most days at around 4pm and had some anyway. Just call me a sad addict; I don't care.)

If money's an issue, consider volunteering Some centres – these tend to be more ashram-style – offer discounted rates to individuals who offer to cook or clean up. You may find a good deal if you're willing to offer a helping hand.

There's no 'right time' for a yoga holiday There's only the right time for you. There are always yoga holidays on offer, near and far. After organising my stepdaughter's wedding, I woke up next morning seriously in need of a yoga vacation and Googled the dates I could go – several options came up. I ended up at a fantastic and very affordable retreat in Abruzzo, Italy – the Shanti Centre (see page 221), and the serendipity worked just fine.

Look at a map Google a map of the destination before booking, if you can, and look very, very closely: there is one thing that a website will never tell you and that is how close your retreat/hotel/ashram is to a major or noisy road. And that can do more to damage your pleasure of being there than almost anything. I once went on a yoga retreat where the traffic noise was a real issue, and will never make that mistake again. So also look whether the venue is close to an airport. That's good in terms of transfers, but if it's a very busy airport you may find yourself cursing the air traffic overhead in a rather un-yoga-like way.

What about hotels and spas with yoga? You might get lucky. I've been to hotels where the 'visiting' yoga teacher has been fantastic, but in general, these classes can be far less satisfying than a full-on yoga retreat. The reason? They're as likely to have to cater to unfit seventy-somethings who haven't touched their toes in a couple of decades as flexible twenty-somethings – and so classes have a 'lowest common denominator' factor, in my experience, and are not particularly challenging. Spas with yoga thrown in are a bit better, I've found, but my real preference would be for a retreat in a location where yoga or meditation is the sole focus of the destination, rather than a trendy 'bolt-on'.

Very importantly, if you book a holiday at a general hotel which

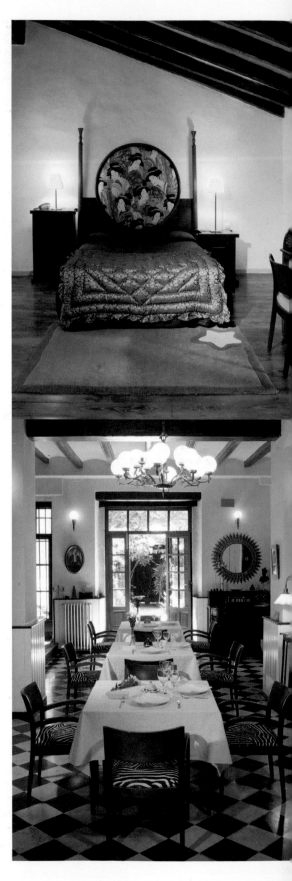

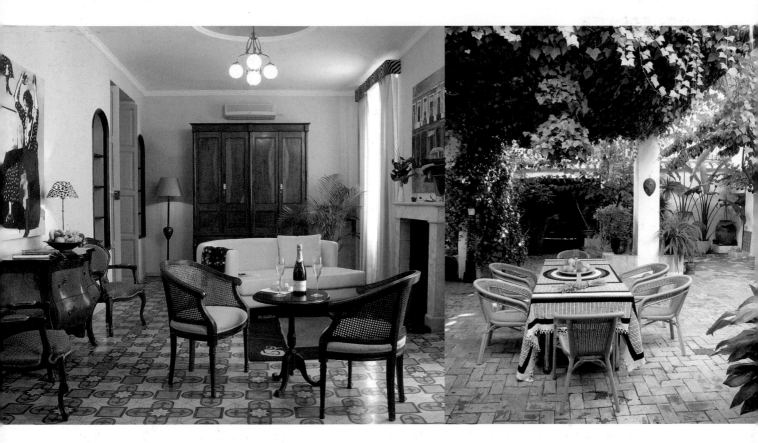

says it offers yoga classes do contact them and make sure that the class is still running. I have twice booked hotels where yoga classes were featured on the website, only to arrive and find that it was the wrong season, or the yoga teacher quit and they hadn't replaced him. Be aware that hotel websites are often seriously out of date – something listed on a site may no longer be on offer.

What to pack? I like the 'wherever I lay my mat, that's my home' approach, so I would recommend packing your own mat. Ditto a large pashmina shawl for relaxation. If you have particular (non-bulky) 'props' that you feel are essential to your practice (a yoga strap, for instance), you might want to consider taking that along. I pack back copies of yoga magazines that I haven't got round to reading, and then leave them behind for other students to enjoy. Try to leave your computer at home and keep your phone switched off: a retreat is a rare and precious chance to unplug from life back home, and immerse yourself in the true spirit of yoga. Which is hard, when your phone's beeping at you. If you rely on your phone to let you know the time of day or wake you up, pack a good, old-fashioned watch or alarm clock instead, so that you're not late for meals or class.

All these photos come from the more luxurious end of the spectrum

Unless there are lots of outings and outdoor activities on offer, you'll probably need fewer clothes than you think. Pack a couple of yoga outfits (and a cardigan/shawl for layering in the cooler evenings), socks (in case your feet get cold in relaxation pose), and a few separates that can be mixed up in the evenings. Good walking shoes are usually handy, plus a swimsuit – and do ask whether beach towels are provided, if there's a pool or a beach nearby (they often aren't).

Remember, it's your vacation On some yoga holidays, participation in all the activities is considered mandatory and there's no real chance to duck out except to fake a headache. Others take a more relaxed view. You don't want to find you've got to join in more than you want to: it can make you feel resentful and grouchy. My 'dream' yoga vacation is 90 minutes practice in the morning and the same later on, with a meditation session, the chance of a good walk and a massage, before an early dinner and deep, deep sleep. But yours might be quite different. Try to get it right before you book by ensuring any questions you may have about the activities are answered.

211

MY TOP YOGA DESTINATIONS

I like to use a UK-based website called Lotus Journeys (www.lotusjourneys.com) which always has a terrific range of yoga holidays on offer. (I have to declare an interest here: Zoe Stebbing, who runs Lotus Journeys, is a relation. But even if she wasn't, I'd turn to this specialist travel agent first, when looking for my next yoga vacation.) For US-based or international retreats, the www.yogajournal.com website is a fantastic resource.

Como Shambhala, Parrot Cay, Turks and Caicos
If you ever, ever have the chance to visit a Como Shambhala hotel, leap at it. This is on a private island in the Caribbean that I was lucky enough to be taken to for 'work': ultra-luxurious, totally secluded, with an open-sided yoga platform overlooking powder-white beaches and classic turquoise Caribbean seascapes. This is a true money-no-object destination, but if money is no object, I can't think of anywhere more perfect to practise yoga. And the standard of teaching is fantastic.
• www.parrotcay.como.bz

Shanti Centre, Abruzzo, Italy
This is at the opposite end of the price spectrum from Parrot Cay, for sure, but Stephanie Shanti and her husband run a busy programme of yoga workshops at their house, often with talented visiting yoga teachers, or taught by Stephanie herself. There are a couple of single rooms as well as doubles, the food is fantastic, and there's a small pool and a sauna. I had a fantastic week of detox and yoga here; just what the doctor ordered (especially the beach-yoga day trip!). Stephanie also offers massage and is one of the best Thai masseurs I've ever been stretched by (and that is saying something).
• www.shanticentre.com

Desa Seni, Canggu, Bali
For a lot of reasons (including friends' recommendations), this is absolutely next on my yoga 'wish list': an eco-friendly village resort in the Balinese countryside, based in antique wooden houses dotted around the 'village' that have been beautifully refurbished and have a serious comfort factor. There's a very wide range of yoga classes on the menu (Kundalini, Anusara, Hatha, Astanga – for explanations of the styles, see pages 32–4). Ubud may be the traditional Balinese destination for yoga (as seen in the Julia Roberts' movie *Eat Pray Love*) with a gazillion classes and retreats on offer, but Canggu is more of a barefoot 'country retreat' setting. I have a special 'Desa Seni piggy bank' on the go.
• www.desaseni.com

Kripalu Center for Yoga and Health, Lenox, Massachusetts, USA
Set in the former estate of steel baron Andrew Carnegie, this might be regarded as a more 'hippy-dippy' yoga retreat, if you like, but it has made the transition from being a 'guru-led' destination to a contemporary well-being retreat, offering a vast range of 'wellness' programmes (many of them unique, such as how to deal with Parkinson's or diabetes) together with an extensive yoga-workshop

calendar. A more stunning setting for your yoga – it's in the Berkshires, which are heavily wooded and with plentiful lakes – is hard to imagine, and just about any yoga teacher who's anyone in the States teaches here at some point.
• www.kripalu.org

Oxen Hoath, Tonbridge, Kent, UK
The advantage of a yoga workshop on your doorstep (albeit far enough away to keep you from the urge to open your mail or stay on top of your laundry) cannot be underestimated, and this beautiful former country house is a hop, skip and a jump away from my home. Regular weekend retreats run here – around six a year – and you can build your own personalised programme of two treatments and a class, or two classes and a treatment, or three classes, for a truly 'bespoke' mini-break. Delicious food and organic wine is served. (As one comment on the website observed, 'Good to find a retreat with a bar.') Treatments include Indian Head Massage, organic spa facials, aromatherapy and shiatsu. The style is slightly 'great-aunt's country house', rather than luxe or 'eco', but there are 28 bedrooms including some singles, and most have their own bathrooms. Personally, I love the 'customised' approach of Oxen Hoath, although they also have a great programme of visiting teachers.
• www.oxenhoath.co.uk

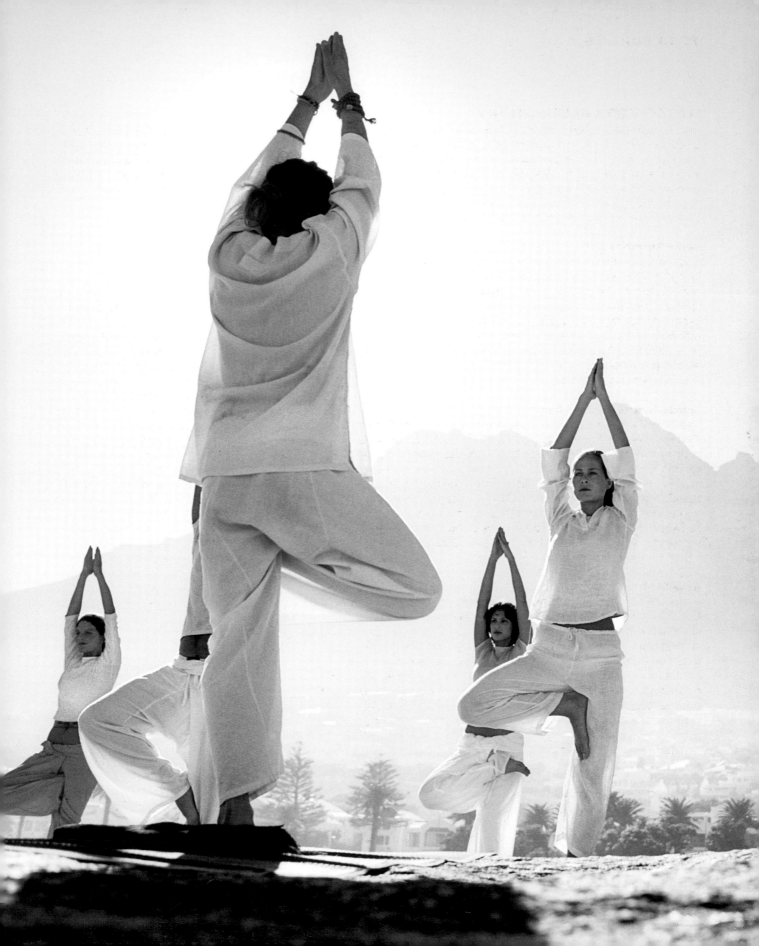

JO FOLEY'S YOGA GETAWAYS

Jo is a globetrotting spa expert and author of *Great Spa Escapes: The Definitive Guide to the Best Spas in the World*.

Ananda in the Himalayas 'My favourite all time yoga location. And it really is the perfect location - in the foothills of the world's most magical mountain range overlooking the valley of the Ganges, and the pilgrim town (Rishikesh) where they claim yoga was born. However, in the clear light and pure air of the early morning the spiritual does take over from the physical. Classes are held in the natural amphitheatre, in the main hall of the old summer palace or in the marble pillared music pavilion with its painted ceiling and glorious views. Where else is better for a sun salutation?'
• www.anandaspa.com

Uma Ubud 'A chic little hideaway on the edge of Bali's cultural capital, Ubud, and part of the Christina Ong stable of hotels from London's Metropolitan to Parrot Cay in the Caribbean. Mrs O is a yoga fanatic and combs the world for the best teachers whom she then inveigles to give week-long retreats at her properties. This is the smallest and sweetest with a yoga pavilion which hangs over the Tjampuhan Valley and is surrounded by jungle, so the only sounds are that of birdsong and the rustle of leaves. No need to wait for a visiting guru: all Ong's yoga teachers are special – head for the boutique too as her yoga clothes are some of the best you will find.'
• www.uma.ubud.como.bz

Swaswara 'The very name, translated from the Sanskrit, means the sound of the self – is a small retreat in the state of Karnataka in India. Just 24 rustic cottages built in local style set among gardens, edged by a lagoon and overlooking a beach called Om. Each day several different types of yoga are on offer from traditional Hatha, through to Astanga, from Laughing to Yoga Nidra plus a number of classes in meditation and Pranayama. Join a class in the circular wooden pavilion and try to stay awake during your Yoga Nidra...otherwise take a private lesson in the open air overlooking the curved golden beach. Find time for some Ayurvedic treatments and a visit to Gorkana, a pilgrim town nearby.'
• www.swaswara.com

Umaid Bhawan Palace in Jodhpur 'The grandest yoga classes can be taken in your own private suite at this hotel. Better still opt for one of the royal suites where you get your own yoga room and the sole attention of Ekraj, the yoga master. He will monitor everything you do and correct and adapt as you progress. Best of all he will follow it up with e-mail reminders and drawings to keep you on the straight and narrow, not to mention supple and bendy. This was the last palace built in India before independence and has the most glamorous circular swimming pool surrounded by Zodiac signs and an Ayurvedic spa – go visit in between yoga classes.'
• www.umaidbhawan.com

Maxine Tobias 'Often it is the yoga teacher rather than the place that begs you to join in. Maxine Tobias is one such teacher and for almost 40 years her studio in London has been a breeding ground for yoga students and devotees. She also holds occasional retreats in rather grand houses along the Eastern Med or the occasional yacht. A tiny tyrant with a rigorous eye for detail, this Iyengar practitioner is regarded as one of the best teachers in the land. Now in her mid-60s she is dedicated to ageless ageing with yoga as its main tool. See her and believe.'
• www.chelseayoga.com

In:Spa Retreats 'In:Spa organise week-long wellness retreats in some of the most beautiful private houses in Marrakech, southern Spain and Provence, taking their own team of trainers, masseurs and yoga teachers along. Jean Hall is one of those yoga teachers who is as inspired as she is inspiring. She also has endless patience and endless kindness with beginners. There is something magical about a yoga class on a rooftop in Marrakech in the early morning or in the shade of an olive grove in late afternoon. Find her dates on the website.'
• www.inspa-retreats.com

Often it is the yoga teacher rather than the place that begs you to join in

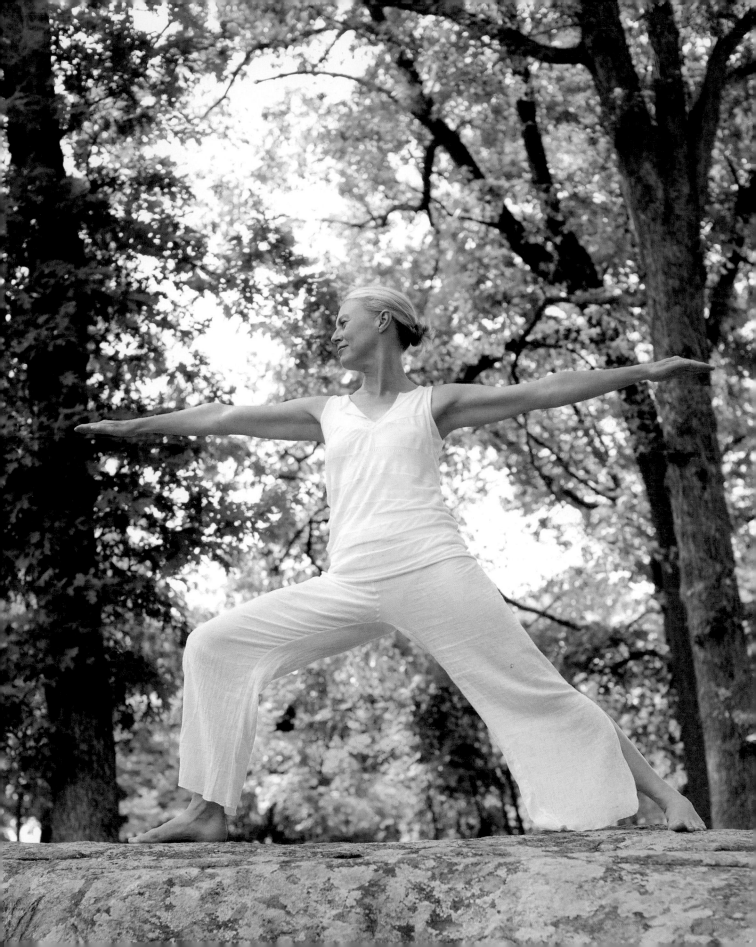

KATHY PHILLIPS'S YOGA RECOMMENDATIONS

Kathy travels a great deal as creator of the This Works aromatherapeutic skincare and bodycare range, and in her role for Condé Nast Asia. A qualified yoga instructor herself, Kathy says, 'To be honest, I would only go somewhere where I knew that there was going to be an inspiring teacher. For me it's all about the teacher and not about the experience of a retreat. With that in mind, the listings here include some teachers who occasionally give intensive classes and workshops as well as retreats that I would recommend.'

Chloe Freemantle weekend retreats at Highgreen Manor, Hexham, Northumberland, UK
Chloe is my teacher and she offers long weekends at Highgreen Manor, a Scottish baronial extravaganza at the centre of an estate that extends over 5,000 acres of moorland. The groups are small, the setting simple but beautiful, and the teaching great.
• www.highgreen-arts.co.uk/Courses

Gurmukh Kaur Kalsa, Golden Bridge Yoga, New York, and Los Angeles, California, USA
A very spiritual and genuine teacher, Gurmukh is co-founder and director of Golden Bridge. The centre offers over 100 classes per week in Kundalini and Hatha yoga taught by many experienced teachers as part of a yoga community that also offers a wellness centre, organic café and yoga marketplace.
• http://la.goldenbridgeyoga.com

Burgs The Art of Meditation retreats, various UK venues
I have done a week of silence on a retreat with Burgs and he is a very special teacher – but this was not luxurious! His teaching style draws on a wide range of influences from his studies of healing meditation practices in Bali, Qigong with Taoist teachers in Asia, and meditation in Burma.
• http://theartofmeditation.org

Simon Low Simon has been teaching for a very long time, which is quite important to me as a recommendation. He is principal of The Yoga Academy and co-founder of Triyoga in London's Primrose Hill, and is known for his innovative 'Yin and Yang' yoga practices. He offers yoga holidays, residential weekends, classes and workshops both in the UK and in Spain, Turkey, India and Thailand.
• www.simonlow.com

Amy Redler Trained by my own teachers, including Mary Stewart, and known for her Thai yoga massage, Amy is a very good yoga teacher and leads workshops and courses in London. She offers annual vacation courses in places such as Italy and Thailand.
• www.kailashcentre.org/amy-redler.html

Kofi Busia A senior Iyengar yoga teacher, Kofi was one of my teachers early on. He is exceptional. Currently based in Santa Cruz, California, he offers yoga workshops and intensives across the US.
• www.kofibusia.com

HIT THE MAT WHEREVER YOU GO

When I travel on business now, I always Google beforehand to find a local yoga class that fits with my schedule. Not long ago I found myself on the mat in San Diego for a 6am 'daybreak' class, which was about as perfect for a jet-lagged traveller from the UK as it's possible to get.

I could go on and on about the joys of dipping into and out of yoga classes abroad. They make you feel like a local, not a tourist, and are a great way to meet people who live and work in the neighbourhood. After that 6am San Diego class, a fellow student took me on a walking tour of the nearby streets, pointing out landmarks and giving me recommendations which simply weren't in any guidebook.

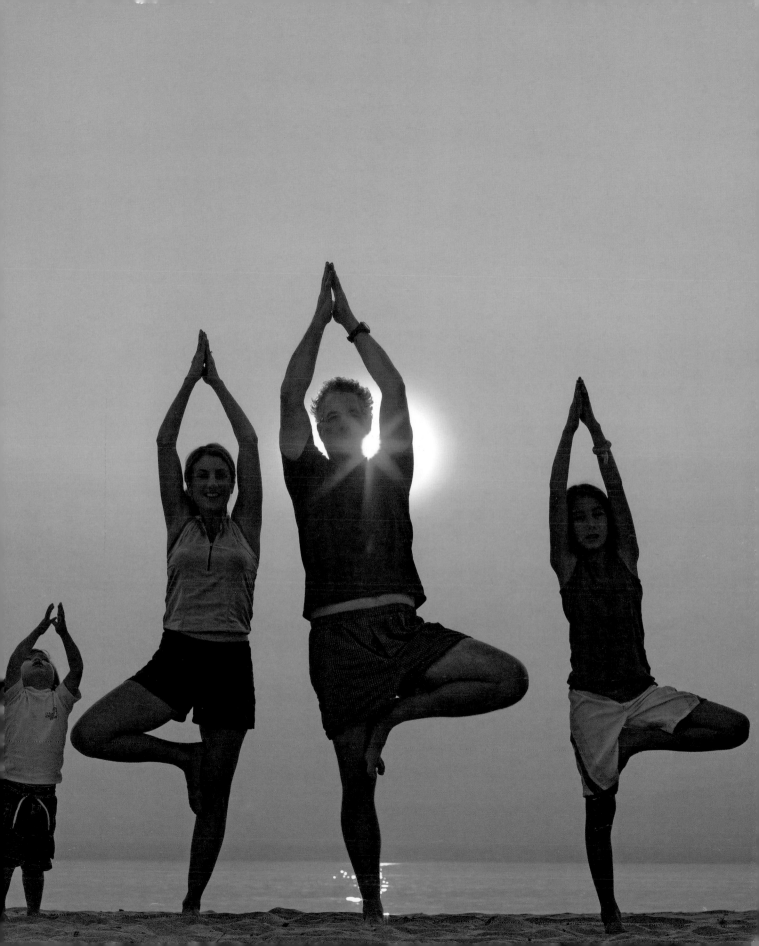

GLOSSARY

YOGA HAS ITS OWN LANGUAGE, Sanskrit, an ancient Indian language considered to be sacred. Some teachers use the original Sanskrit names for postures, which can be incredibly confusing. And some people find it irritating – I have one friend who bristles when our teacher uses Sanskrit names for poses, though I have pointed out that she doesn't think twice about ordering a cappuccino or a macchiato....

Throughout this book I have used the English name first, then the Sanskrit name if there is one (some of the poses here are not found in the classical repertoire and so don't have a name). Here is a cribsheet for most of the postures (with pronunciations in brackets). If you go to a class where the teacher uses Sanskrit and you find it hard to follow the instructions, never feel inhibited about asking for the names of the postures in English, too. At this stage in life we are all surely past the point of shyness, and the last thing a yoga class should be about is stressing over not understanding what you're meant to be doing.

(NB In the list on the right, place the emphasis on the syllables in italics.)

JO'S YOGA STUDIO IS AT:
The Wellington Centre
44 Wellington Square
Hastings
East Sussex
TN34 1PN
01424 442520
www.thewellingtoncentre.com

YOGA DIRECTORY
Follow Jo Fairley's yoga news on
Twitter: **@yoga4lifebook**
Follow Jo on Twitter: **@jojosams**

Visit **www.yogaforlifebook.com**
for more information

Adho Mukha Svanasana – **Downward-facing Dog Pose**
  (*AH-doh MOO-kuh shvah-NAHS-ah-nuh*)
Ananda Balasana - **Happy Baby Pose**
  (*Ann-AN-dah bal-AHS-ah-nuh*)
Baddha Konasana – **Cobbler Pose** (*BAW-dah con-NAHS-ah-nuh*)
Balasana – **Child Pose** (*Bal-AHS-ah-nuh*)
Bharadvajasana – **Simple Twist** (*Bah-ROD-va-JAHS- ah-nuh*)
Bhujangasana – **Cobra Pose** (*Boo-jan-GAHS-ah-nuh*)
Dandasana – **Staff Pose** (*Dan-DAHS-ah-nuh*)
Eka Pada Adho Mukha Svanasana –
  One-legged Downward-facing Dog Pose
  (*EK-uh- PAW-duh AH-doh MOO-kuh shvah-NAHS- ah-nuh*)
Garudasana – **Eagle Pose** (*Gah-roo-DAHS-ah-nuh*)
Kapotasana - **Pigeon Pose** (*KAH-put-AHS-ah-nuh*)
Marjari Asana – **Cat Pose** (*Mah-JAH-ree AHS-ah-nuh*)
Nadi Shodhana Pranayama – **Alternate-nostril Breathing**
  (*Nah-dee Sho-DAH-nah pra-nah-YAH-mah*)
Padangusthasana – **Big Toe Pose** (*POD-un-goos-TAHS-ah-nuh*)
Paschimottanasana – **Seated Forward Bend**
  (*POSH-ee moh-tun-AHS-ah-nuh*)
Prasarita Padottanasana – **Wide-legged Forward Bend**
  (*Pra-SA-rita pa-dot-ANAHS-ah-nuh*)
Salamba Bhujangasana – **Sphinx Pose**
  (*Sah-LAM-bah Boo-jan-GAHS-ah-nuh*)
Salamba Sarvangasana – **Supported Shoulderstand**
  (*Sah-LAM-ba Shar-van-GAHS-ah-nuh*)
Savasana – **Corpse Pose** (*Shah-VAHS-ah-nuh*)
Setu Bandha Sarvangasana – **Bridge Pose**
  (*SET-too BAWN-duh sar-van-GOSS-ah-nuh*)
Sukhasana – **Easy Pose** (*Sook-AH-sah-nuh*)
Tadasana – **Mountain Pose** (*Tah-DAH-sah-nuh*)
Ujjayi Pranayama – **Ocean Breath** (*Ooh-JAI pra-nah-YAH-mah*)
Urdhva Hastasana in Tadasana –
  Mountain Pose with Arms Overhead
  (*Oord-VAH-hahs-TAHS-ah-nuh*)
Urdhva Mukha Svanasana – **Upward-facing Dog Pose**
  (*OORD-vah MOO-kuh shvah-NAHS-ah-nuh*)
Uttanasana – **Standing Forward Bend** (*Ooh-tah-NAHS-ah-nuh*)
Trikonasana – **Triangle Pose** (*Trik-o-NAHS-ah-nuh*)
Viparita Karani – **Legs-up-the-wall Pose**
  (*Vee-pah-REET-uh ka-RAH-nee*)
Virabhadrasana I - **Warrior Pose I** (*Veer-ah-bah-DRAHS-ah-nuh*)
Vrksasana – **Tree Pose** (*Vrik-SHAHS-ah-nuh*)

YOGA RESOURSES

STYLES OF YOGA

GENERAL ... An international 'umbrella' site for classes globally is www.yogafinder.com
UK www.yoga-magazine.net
lists many UK teachers across different styles of yoga.
US www.yogajournal.com has an excellent directory where you can search by Zip Code for teachers, or browse by style/ US State. The following sections feature specific sites for different styles of yoga, but the Yoga Journal site is a great short-cut, too. Also visit
www.americanyogaassociation.org
AUSTRALIA www.findyoga.com.au
offers the largest directory of classes, teachers and events
NEW ZEALAND www.iyta.org.nz
SOUTH AFRICA www.vedicvista.co.za
lists Hatha yoga schools and teachers across South Africa

ANUSARA
UK Bridget Woods Kramer is the UK's Anusara representative;
www.bridgetwoodskramer.com
US/WORLDWIDE (including AUSTRALIA and SOUTH AFRICA)
www.anusara.com

ASTANGA
UK There is no specific Astanga organisation in the UK but if you Google 'Astanga UK', you can locate many different teachers/centres.
US – visit
www.yogajournal.com/directory/style/ashtanga
AUSTRALIA
Use Google to find the nearest class to you
NEW ZEALAND Use Google to find the nearest class to you
SOUTH AFRICA Use Google to find the nearest class to you

HATHA
UK British Wheel of Yoga
www.bwy.org.uk
US www.yogausa.com
AUSTRALIA – see GENERAL, above
NEW ZEALAND – see GENERAL, above
SOUTH AFRICA - see GENERAL, above

IYENGAR
UK www.iyengaryoga.org.uk
US www.iynaus.org
www.iyengar-yoga.com
AUSTRALIA www.iyengaryoga.asn.au
NEW ZEALAND www.iyengar-yoga.org.nz
SOUTH AFRICA www.bksiyengar.co.za

JIVAMUKTI
UK www.jivamuktiyoga.co.uk
US/WORLDWIDE www.jivamuktiyoga.com

KUNDALINI
UK www.kundaliniyoga.org.uk
US www.kundalini-yoga.us
AUSTRALIA www.kundaliniyoga.com.au
NEW ZEALAND
www.kundaliniyoga-nz.com
SOUTH AFRICA www.kundaliniyoga.co.za

RESTORATIVE
Not an 'official' style of yoga so best to Google for local classes to you.

SCARAVELLI
UK There is no specific Scaravelli yoga organisation although an increasing number of locations offer Scaravelli-inspired yoga classes; use Google to find the nearest to you
US www.vandascaravelliyoga.com
(NB This is not a 'national' Scaravelli organisation but the website of two individual teachers; however, it has useful in-depth info about this style of yoga. Again, use Google – or www.yogajournal.com - to find Scaravelli teachers near you.)

AUSTRALIA www.annacrowley.com is the website of a Melbourne-based Scaravelli teacher with useful links to other practitioners/workshops in Australia
NEW ZEALAND Use Google to find the nearest class to you
SOUTH AFRICA Use Google to find the nearest class to you

SIVANANDA
UK www.sivananda.co.uk
US www.sivananda.org
AUSTRALIA www.sivananda.co.uk/au or see GENERAL, above
NEW ZEALAND www.sivanandayoga.co.nz
SOUTH AFRICA No national organisation so Google to find local classes

VINYASA FLOW
Use Google – or see GENERAL, above - to find local classes

YOGA NIDRA
Use Google – or see GENERAL, above - to find local classes, or use the resources below – CDs and MP3s – to practise this at home.
www.nidrayoga.co.uk (this site offers a free MP3 download of Yoga Nidra)
Yoga Nidra audio practice - visit
www.myyogaonline.com
Drops of Nectar by Shiva Rea (Sound True) features a Yoga Nidra CD
More Yoga Nidra recordings are available for download at the iTunes Store **(www.apple.com/itunes)**
Yoga Nidra Relaxation – Rest Peacefully & Manage Sleep Disorders Through Self-Hypnoses: **Guided Meditation & Yoga Nidra with Dr. Siddharth Ashvin Shah.**
Drops of Nectar by Shiva Rea (also on iTunes)

DIRECTORY

YOGA KIT
CLOTHING
prAna - www.prana.com
Gossypium - www.gossypium.co.uk
Sweaty Betty – www.sweatybetty.co.uk

MATS/BLOCKS/ACCESSORIES
(NB prAna mats, which I particularly rate, are also now available via Amazon)
UK www.yogamatters.com
www.barefootyoga.com
www.glowgetter.co.uk
US www.yogamad.com
www.prana.com
www.yogamats-bags.com
is a good 'umbrella' site for equipment
AUSTRALIA www.yogagear.net.au
www.iyogaprops.com.au
www.mat-tastic.com.au
NEW ZEALAND
www.yogasupplies.co.nz
www.yoga.co.nz
www.ecoyogastore.co.nz

EYE PILLOWS
UK www.bwy-shop.co.uk
US www.pillowcompany.com
AUSTRALIA www.lotusskincare.com.au
NEW ZEALAND www.ecoyogastore.co.nz

INCENSE
Himalaya Spa incense is available from
www.glowgetter.co.uk
(they ship worldwide)

MEDITATION
www.kundaliniresearchinstitute.org
Australian Bush Flower Essences -
UK www.victoriahealth.com and
www.baldwins.co.uk

See **YOGA BOOKSHELF** for Meditation books

INTERNATIONAL - visit
www.ausflowers.com.au
for international distributors

YOGA TRAVEL WEBSITES
www.yogajournal.com
www.destinationyoga.co.uk
www.lotusjourneys.com
www.thebaoli.com
www.retreatsonline.com
www.yogafinder.com

HAPPY YOGA HOLIDAYS

Como Shambhala, Turks & Caicos –
www.comoshambhala.como.bz
and www.parrotcay.como.bz
Shanti Centre, Abruzzo, Italy –
www.shanticentre.com
Desa Seni, Bali –
www.desaseni.com
Kripalu, Massachusetts, USA –
www.kripalu.org
Oxon Hoath, Kent, UK –
www.oxonhoath.co.uk

KATHY PHILLIPS'S RECOMMENDATIONS

Chloe Fremantle –
chloeblegvad@btinternet.com
Gurmukh – www.gurmukh.com
The Art of Meditation with Burgs –
www.theartofmeditation.org
Simon Low - www.simonlow.com
Amy Redler – see
www.kailashcentre.org
Kofi Busia – www.kofibusia.com

JO FOLEY'S RECOMMENDATIONS

Ananda www.anandaspa.com
Uma Ubud www.uma.ubud.como.bz
Swaswara www.swaswara.com
Umaid Bhawan Palace
www.umaidbhawan.com
Maxine Tobias www.chelseayoga.com
In:spa www.inspa-retreats.com

SOME GREAT YOGA WEBSITES

www.yogajournal.com
www.kineticvigilantes.com
www.myyogaonline.com
www.theyogalunchbox.co.nz
www.yogapages.co.uk
www.abc-of-yoga.com
www.marianne-elliott.com

EAT YOUR YOGA

The Synergy Company Pure Synergy –
UK www.glowgetter.co.uk
US AND INTERNATIONAL
www.thesynergycompany.com
Vegetarian Food Pyramid –
www.vegetariannutrition.org
(go to RESOURCES)
See also **YOGA BOOKSHELF**

YOGA BOOKSHELF

Some of these are out-of-print but thanks to the glories of the internet, can still usually be sourced via
www.amazon.com or www.abebooks.com

AYURVEDA MADE SIMPLE: An Easy-to-follow Guide to the Ancient System of Health and Diet by Body Type by Sally Morningstar *(Southwater)*

BE HERE NOW by Ram Dass *(Crown Publications)*

BOOST YOUR VITALITY WITH AYURVEDA by Sarah Lie *(Teach Yourself books)*

BREATHWALK: Breathing Your Way to a Revitalized Body, Mind & Spirit by Gurucharan Singh Khalsa and Yogi Bhajan *(Broadway Books)*

FOOD FOR THE SOUL by Manuela Dun Mascetti and Arunima Borthwick *(New Leaf)*

GENTLE YOGA FOR OSTEOPOROSIS by Laurie Sanford *(Hatherleigh Press)*

GREAT SPA ESCAPES: The Definitive Guide to the Best Spas in the World by Jo Foley *(Daikini Books)*

GUIDED MINDFULNESS MEDITATION by Jon Kabat-Zinn *(Sounds True Inc.)*

INNER BALANCE: Eleven Guided Meditations *(New Balance)*

INTUITIVE EATING: A Revolutionary Programme That Works by Evelyn Tribole and Elyse Resch *(St. Martin's Griffin)*

IYENGAR YOGA: Classic Postures for Mind, Body and Spirit by Judy Smith *(Southwater)*

LIGHT ON YOGA by B.K.S. Iyengar *(Thorsons)*

LIVING YOGA: Creating a Life Practice by Christy Turlington *(Penguin)*

MEDITATION FOR BEGINNERS by Jack Kornfield *(Bantam)*

MEDITATION FOR DUMMIES by Dean Ornish MD and Stephan Bodian *(John Wiley & Sons)*

MINDLESS EATING: Why We Eat More Than We Think by Brian Wansink *(Hay House)*

STILL HERE: Embracing Aging, Changing and Dying by Ram Dass *(Riverhead Books)*

THE HEALTHY KITCHEN by Andrew Weil, M.D. and Rosie Daly *(Knopf)*

THE MACROBIOTIC BROWN RICE COOKBOOK by Craig Sams *(Inner Traditions)*

THE MOOSEWOOD RESTAURANT COOKING FOR HEALTH by Mollie Katzen *(Simon Spotlight Entertainment)*

THE SACRED KITCHEN: Higher Consciousness Cooking for Health and Wholeness by Robin Robertson and Jon Robertson *(New World Library)*

THE SPIRIT OF YOGA by Kathy Phillips *(Hachette)*

THE YOGA OF BREATH: A Step-by-Step Guide to Pranayama by Richard Rosen

YOGA – A Gem for Women by Geeta S. Iyengar *(Timeless Books)*

YOGA AS MEDICINE by Timothy McCall, M.D. *(A Yoga Journal Book)*

YOGA FOR HEALTHY KNEES by Sandy Blaine *(Rodmell Press)*

YOGA FOR OSTEOPOROSIS: The Complete Guide by Loren Fishman *(W.W. Norton & Co.)*

YOGA FOR WOMEN AT MIDLIFE AND BEYOND by Pat Shapiro *(Sun Stone Press)*

YOGI IN THE KITCHEN by Elaine Gavalas *(Avery)*

INDEX

ACKNOWLEDGEMENTS

There are many individuals I'd like to thank for their help – or their inspiration – writing this book: the talented 'East Sussex team' of **Claire Richardson** (photographer) and **Debi Angel** (designer and tassel-tweaker); Claire's photographic assistants **Amy Barton** and **Kristy Noble**; **Vicky Orchard** from Kyle Books (editor and yoga-gear-sourcer extraordinaire); **Stuart MacKay** from Beyond Hope for providing the prAna gear for our models (www.beyondhope.co.uk); **David Edmunds** (for helping to ferry props) and **Amy Eason** (general all-round wonderfulness); **Sarah Stacey** (my ever-patient *Beauty Bible* co-author); **Kay McCauley** (wonder-agent) and **Kyle Cathie** (ever-brilliant publisher); **Chris Elam** for his diligent reading; **Emma Jane Frost** for the mouthwatering food styling; **Kathy Phillips** and **Jo Foley** for their yoga travel suggestions; all the teachers at **The Wellington Centre** (www.thewellingtoncentre. com); **Glenda Petersen** for relocating her Pilates classes to allow us to shoot in the yoga studio; our wonderful yogis, photographed for the book – **Alex**, **Judy**, **Nicola**, **Simon** and **Cindy** – and not forgetting the boys at **Waterfalls Café** in Hastings for the best shoot lunches ever. Huge appreciation to Simon Low for his wonderful foreword – who could have guessed the paths we'd take all those years ago...? And, as always, **Craig Sams**, who shared my Wellington Centre dream – and is the best supporter and partner in life I could ever wish for.